FITNESS FOR EVERY BODY

LINDA GARRISON
Mt. San Antonio College

ANN K. READ
Fullerton College

 Mayfield Publishing Company

Library of Congress Catalog Card Number: 79-91831
International Standard Book Number: 0-87484-444-4

Manufactured in the United States of America
Mayfield Publishing Company
285 Hamilton Avenue, Palo Alto, California 94301

This book was set in Optima with display type in Korinna Italic by
Viking Typographics and was printed and bound by the George Banta
Company. Sponsoring editor was C. Lansing Hays, Maggie Cutler
supervised editing, and Gene Tanke was manuscript editor. Book design is by Nancy Sears, page make up by Pat Rogondino, and artwork
by Carole Etow. Michelle Hogan supervised production. The cover
design is by Joan Brown.

CONTENTS

PREFACE

Exercise and nutrition are of growing interest to modern men and women in their search for health, physical fitness, and a more attractive body. As a result of this interest, a great number of individuals and groups are realizing a tremendous profit. However, the growing amount of misinformation concerning exercise, beauty, health, and physical fitness is alarming, and in some cases actually dangerous. We owe it to ourselves to become more knowledgeable in these areas.

This book, then, is an attempt to educate: to present accurate knowledge in the areas of nutrition and exercise and to present information for both sexes. Although primarily designed as a text for use in physical education classes at the college level, the authors hope that this book will also be of interest to adults of all ages, whether or not they are engaged in formal education.

The task of condensing so much needed information into so small a capsule has not been simple; at times, indeed, it seemed impossible. But now that we have finished the book, we feel that we have learned a lot from the experience of writing it. And, we hope that you, the reader, will learn from, and enjoy, the experience of reading it.

A book is never completed by authors alone, and many persons helped us along the way. We especially want to thank Diana Zigars, who gave us ideas and helped prepare initial illustrative material; Gayle Gess of Fullerton College, for her critical review of the nutrition materials; and our publisher, editors, illustrator, and the staff of Mayfield Publishing Company for their various efforts, as well as for their patience and understanding. In addition we wish to express our appreciation to the authors and publishers who allowed us to make use of their published material. Finally, we thank the following reviewers who gave us so many helpful comments: Nancy Anderson of Wartburg College, Harry P. DuVal of Indiana University, Joe Hicks of Long Beach City College, Clair Jennett of San Jose State University, Nancy J. Mikleton of Clackamas Community College, Walt Rilliet of Skyline College, and William C. Savage of Boston University.

1 | *FINDING FITNESS IN TODAY'S WORLD*

It is interesting to note that among the healthiest and most long-lived people on earth are the Abkhansian peasants who reside in the rural farming communities of Russia. The apparent key to their youth and vigor is their way of life, which is simple and close to nature.[1] They are vigorous and active into their declining years; their diet is quite simple, and yet more nutritious than that of their more civilized counterparts; and they seem to have a more relaxed way of living.

By contrast, our American standard of living has become a detriment to our overall health. On one hand, machines and "labor-saving" devices increasingly dominate our lifestyle, replacing physical activity. How do you react when an elevator is not working and you have to climb the stairs, or when you leave your house to find that your car has a flat tire?

Electric golf carts, snowmobiles, dune buggies, and motorbikes make even our physical exercise less taxing. And of course there is the television habit; countless hours once spent in outdoor activity are now spent indoors in front of the tube. On the other hand, the mass marketing of prepackaged (and preservative-laden) supermarket items, and of high-calorie fast-food goodies, have made relatively nutrition-poor foods a large part of our diet.

Few of us would actually like to go backward in time to a world without machines or food stores. The alternative is to make more intelligent use of what our culture provides. We must become constantly aware of the price we pay for letting machines make us totally inactive and letting convenience foods impoverish our diet.

COPING WITH OUR ENVIRONMENT

We can learn to cope with our environment in better ways, even though an advancing technology will continue to offer new ways to replace physical labor and change eating habits.

Activity must become a regular part of our lives. Exercise must be planned to fit into busy schedules and bad weather conditions.

> *Ecology is the branch of science concerned with the interrelationship of living organisms and their environment. Within this term it is appropriate to consider both the fitness of an environment to sustain life and the ability of organisms to tolerate their environment.*
>
> —JEAN MAYER
> *Health*

Adding exercise and nutrition to everyday living is not always easy and pleasant, especially at first. Jogging must sometimes be done in rain or snow, and the convenience of buying high-calorie fast foods must be given up in favor of arranging meals which are low in calories but high in nutrition. The results, however, will be well worth the effort. You will look better and feel better in just a few weeks after beginning the health program we describe.

THE STEPS TOWARD CHANGE

We are creatures of habit, and habits are difficult to give up. To begin making desired changes, we must do some inner searching and assessment and begin retraining ourselves in the following areas.

DEVELOPING AWARENESS   Becoming more aware of yourself is one of the keys to success in changing habits. Habits are established by the repetition of behavior, so making behavioral changes becomes very important. In order to make such changes, you must know yourself and become aware of your every action. Developing awareness is the essential first step toward gaining conscious control of behavior.

ANALYZING BEHAVIOR   Behavior must be analyzed before it can be changed. You must understand why you act the way you do. What prompts you to act in certain ways, and how closely are these related to your lifestyle? Consider your lifestyle as a set of patterns established by your behavior. Try to identify the behavioral patterns that cause problems, and then try to determine why they exist.

Many unproductive behavior patterns are the outcome of a negative self-image.[2] A negative self-image is accompanied by a lack of self-confidence, feelings of inadequacy, and in many cases by a feeling of being unloved. In order to develop the motivation to change behavioral patterns, you must work on your self-image. "Almost without exception, individuals who have the negative self-image problem are in reality, individuals of good capability and are objectively very adequate."[3] Continue the improvement of your self-image by repeating that you are important and have unique talents or other assets. Sometimes it helps to write down your advantages, assets, and talents.

> *You are not born with a self-image; you acquire one. The fact that a person is responsible for his actions is a part of his self-image. Because this is so, self-control and self-direction accompany a healthy self-concept. An important aspect of your self-image is your frame of reference. If you have an unrealistic or defective frame of reference, your view of yourself will be distorted.*
>
> —ANN ELLENSON
> *Human Relations*

Your level of motivation will determine your readiness to begin making behavioral changes. Knowledge and understanding are very important to motivation. If you are to change your level of health and physical well-being, you must first recognize that there are problems, and then become convinced that they need to be solved.

GOAL SETTING   The next step is to determine the changes that must occur in order to reach the desired results. As problem areas are analyzed, a desired result (a goal) should be set. After all goals have been set, look at them in terms of time. Divide them into two categories: short-term and long-term goals. Then set a tentative time schedule for their accomplishment. Short-term goals are those that can probably be met in a number of days or weeks, whereas long-term goals may take months or even years to accomplish. As you begin to reach your first short-term goals, you will enjoy feelings of success and growth that will carry you forward.

EVALUATION   Goals should be evaluated periodically. The evaluation should take into account changes in your lifestyle as well as the changes you have made in yourself. Some goals will have been met, and others will need to be redefined. Some goals may have been unrealistic or undesirable, and will need to be changed. In the beginning, evaluations should take place every other month, and later at yearly intervals.

> *To winners, time is precious. Winners don't kill it, but live it here and now. Living in the now does not mean that winners foolishly ignore their own past history or fail to prepare for the future. Rather, winners know their past, are aware and alive in the present, and look forward to the future.*
>
> —JAMES and JONGEWARD
> *Born to Win*

FOLLOWING YOUR NEW LIFESTYLE

Concentration and self-discipline are two of the keys to success in almost any plan of action. Concentration and self-discipline help you to persevere. These are not innate powers, but rather ones that must be learned and practiced. Your ability to resist temptation will depend on your self-discipline and your power to concentrate on the goals you have set. In the words of Carl Rogers, "To be responsibly self-directing means that one chooses and then learns from the consequences."[4]

You control your future, and you have the opportunity to pursue the type of lifestyle that will give you the future you want. Use the material in the following chapters to help you reach your goals.

Notes
1. Lawrence E. Lamb, *Stay Youthful and Fit* (New York: Harper and Row Publishers, 1974), pp. 4–5.
2. Abraham J. Twerski, *Like Yourself* (Englewood Cliffs: Prentice-Hall, Inc., 1978), p. 7.
3. *Ibid.*, pp. 6–7.
4. Carl R. Rogers, *On Becoming a Person* (Boston: Houghton Mifflin Company, 1961), p. 171.

2 | *MUSCLES AND CURVES*

This era of changing sex roles has caused us to question whether the observed differences between men and women are learned or inherent.[1] We are aware that even today little boys and little girls are still treated differently. From the minute a newborn baby girl is wrapped in a pink blanket and her brother in a blue one, the two children are treated differently.[2] Are there basic physiological differences with which we should be concerned? And how do these differences relate to activity and physical fitness?

Although there are many physiological differences between men and women, the material presented here will be concerned chiefly with those differences that influence physical activity.

BODY COMPOSITION

Before puberty, the basic physiological differences between boys and girls are insignificant as they relate to physical activity. However, with the onset of puberty (usually between the ages of 10 and 13), the differences do become significant.

When full maturity is reached, the average female is five inches shorter than the average male, thirty to forty pounds lighter in total weight, forty to fifty pounds lighter in lean body weight, and considerably fatter—having 25 versus 15 percent relative body fat.[3] This means that the male is characterized by a stronger, heavier body, because of his higher percentage of muscular tissue and lower percentage of fatty tissue. This also accounts for the difference between the strength-to-weight ratio between men and women and is one of the reasons why on the average men are significantly stronger than women.[4]

> *The differences between the two sexes is one of the important conditions upon which we have built the many varieties of human culture that give human beings dignity and stature.*
>
> —MARGARET MEAD
> *Male and Female*

Another important factor is the difference in the distribution of body fat in men and women. The male has a greater amount of subcutaneous fat in the abdominal and upper regions of the body, while the female carries substantially more fat in the hip and lower regions of the body.[5]

HORMONAL INFLUENCES

Most, if not all, of the basic physiological differences between men and women can be directly related to the secretion of the androgen hormones in the male and the estrogen hormones in the female. Of the androgen hormones, testosterone is so much more abundant and potent than the others that one can consider it to be the single significant hormone responsible for the male hormonal effects.[6] On the other hand, the female hormone, estrogen, primarily seems to be responsible for the female reproductive system.

Testosterone is responsible for the following secondary sexual characteristics that differentiate the male from the female:

1. Faster bone and tissue growth, including stimulated blood flow which causes greater muscular development.
2. Distribution of body hair over the genital organs, on the face, chest, and sometimes the back; more prolific hair growth on other parts of the body; and a decrease in the growth of hair on the top of the head, which when combined with a genetic background for the development of baldness, causes baldness.
3. Greater deposits of protein in the skin, muscles, bones, and other parts of the body, causing a generally larger and more muscular structure.
4. Changes in the larynx resulting in a lower voice.

5. A metabolic rate as much as 15 percent higher.
6. A greater number of red blood cells.[7]

In addition to being responsible for the female reproductive system, the estrogens, including progesterone, share the responsibility for the following secondary sexual characteristics in the female:

1. Greater fatty deposits in the breasts.
2. Broadening of the hips and pelvis.
3. Deposits of greater quantities of fat in the subcutaneous tissues.
4. A period of rapid growth which begins and ends before the male's fast growth-rate period does.
5. Smooth-textured, soft skin.[8]

THE EFFECTS OF CONDITIONING

Although both males and females benefit from exercise, there will be differences in its effect. Women should not be afraid of developing bulky muscles. While strength training does produce large increases in the female's total body strength, it does *not* appear to result in large gains in muscle bulk.[9] This is due to the low level of testosterone in the female.

The male's greater muscle concentration and larger bone size can inhibit his flexibility.[10] Proper conditioning techniques in flexibility exercises can help correct this tendency.

> *How are men and women to think about their maleness and their femaleness in this twentieth century, in which so many of our old ideas must be made new? Have we over-domesticated men, denied their natural adventurousness, tied them down to machines that are after all only glorified spindles and looms, mortars and pestles and digging sticks, all of which were once women's work? Have we cut women off from their natural closeness to their children, taught them to look for a job instead of the touch of a child's hand, for status in a competitive world rather than a unique place by a glowing hearth? In educating women like men, have we done something disastrous to both men and women alike, or have we only taken one further step in the recurrent task of building more and better on our original human nature?*
>
> —MARGARET MEAD
> *Male and Female*

Although it is unlikely that women will ever reach the speed of men at running or swimming short to medium distances, recent studies have shown that the extra percentage of fatty tissue in women makes them ideally suited for long-distance, endurance activities, during which great amounts of stored energy must be available.[11] This characteristic may account for the fact that women seem to excel in long-distance swimming.

Despite the substantial physiological differences between males and females after the onset of puberty, recent studies have suggested that the highly trained female is not greatly different from her highly trained male counterpart.[12] In the past, girls have been excluded from most rigorous physical activities.[13] Girls have been taught to be passive and sedentary, whereas boys have been taught to be aggressive and active. A sedentary lifestyle naturally leads to a deterioration in the level of physical fitness. Therefore, what appear to be dramatic biological differences between the sexes in fact may be more related to cultural and social restrictions placed on the female.[14]

Notes

1. Lenore J. Weitzman, *Sex Role Socialization* (Palo Alto: Mayfield Publishing Company, 1977), p. ix.
2. *Ibid.*, p. 1.
3. Jack H. Wilmore and A. R. Behnke, "An Anthropometric Estimation of Body Density and Lean Body Weight in Young Men," *Journal of Applied Physiology* 27 (1969): 25.
4. Anthony Smith, *The Body* (New York: Avon Books, 1969), pp. 333–37.
5. Jack H. Wilmore, *Athletic Training and Physical Fitness* (Boston: Allyn and Bacon, Inc., 1977), p. 181.
6. Arthur C. Guyton, *Textbook of Medical Physiology,* (Philadelphia: W. B. Saunders Company, 1976), p. 1078.
7. *Ibid.*, pp. 1080–81.
8. *Ibid.*, pp. 1092–93.
9. Wilmore, *Athletic Training,* p. 182.
10. Janet A. Wessel, *Movement Fundamentals* (Englewood Cliffs: Prentice-Hall, Inc., 1970), p. 71.
11. *Ibid.*
12. Wilmore, *Athletic Training,* p. 187.
13. Weitzman, *Sex Role Socialization,* p. 38.
14. Wilmore, *Athletic Training,* p. 187.

3 | NUTRITION

Nutrition is the science of food. Food is essential to one's very existence because it is used to rebuild cells or to build new cells replacing those which the body constantly loses. The body is continually rebuilding; the average red blood cell circulates for only 120 days.[1] Consider the effect of sunburn on the skin, how it blisters and peels, and the build-up of hair in combs and brushes. These are examples of the way the body constantly renews tissue.

The old saying, "You are what you eat," is far more accurate than one would think. The food a person eats contains the nutrients needed to rebuild cells and to aid the body in maintaining a healthy, functioning status. The type and the amount of food consumed affects body size, appearance, disposition, strength, intelligence (learning and retention), stamina, and even length of life.[2]

FROM FOOD TO NUTRIENTS TO YOU

The basic nutrients the body requires can be divided into six classes: water, vitamins, minerals, carbohydrates, protein, and fats.[3] The body will obtain these nutrients from the foods consumed, provided a balanced diet is followed.[4]

Through digestion, the food is broken down into minute particles. Then the process of absorption takes place. During this process the nutrients are transferred from the intestinal wall into the blood and lymph circulation.[5] From this point on the feeding of the body takes place.

Metabolism is the term used to describe the chemical reactions and changes that take place in the cells after absorption.[6] Metabolism is broken-down into *anabolism* and *catabolism*. "Anabolism includes the processes by which the absorbed products of digestion are used to replace body constituents and to form new cellular material for growth."[7] "Catabolism, by contrast, refers to the breaking down of complex substances such as nutrients into simpler substances."[8]

All body processes . . . may be affected by the lack of even one essential nutrient. The synthesis of red blood cells, for example, requires not only iron but also copper, cobalt, fats and carbohydrates, protein, and numerous vitamins. If any of these nutrients is missing from the diet, anemia can result.

— INSEL and ROTH
Health in A Changing Society

Enzymes must be present in the body in order for metabolism to take place. This is where vitamins and minerals play an important role. Respiration is also important in the process of transferring the nutrients to the cells. The respiratory system provides the oxygen necessary for making use of nutrients and provides a method for eliminating waste products. Enzymes help the cell to use the nutrient.

In a complex series of steps, glucose (carbohydrates) and fats are oxidized to release the energy needed for the body's work.[9] Any excess is stored for future use. This is important to know for weight control purposes. Protein is broken down into amino acids, which are used to build and repair cells, to form hormones and enzymes, and as an additional source of energy.[10] Excess protein also becomes adipose tissue (fat). In addition to aiding the production of enzymes, minerals act to regulate body metabolism and acid-base balance.

WATER   Water provides the medium in which nearly all of the body's reactions take place, as well as supplying the means of transporting materials to and from cells—for water surrounds every cell of the body.[11] Although a person can live for a few weeks without food, life can be sustained for only a few days without water. About two thirds of one's body weight consists of water, which must constantly be replenished, at a rate of one to two quarts daily.[12] The importance of water to the body is so great that a loss of only 10 percent will result in severe disorders, and a 20 percent loss can result in death.[13]

VITAMINS AND MINERALS   Vitamins and minerals, as we noted earlier, are important to the digestive process. With few exceptions, a balanced diet will yield the proper vitamins and minerals. Iron is the most common mineral deficiency found in American diets. Young women and pregnant women should be especially aware of this fact and should add an iron supplement to their diet if necessary. This might also be recommended for the weight-conscious, because restricted food intakes tend to provide only small amounts of iron. Vitamins are an entirely different matter. It is most unusual for people who eat a balanced diet to have a vitamin deficiency. In the United States vitamin overdosage is probably a bigger risk than a deficiency.[14] Long-term excess use of some high potency vitamin pills can cause vitamin toxicity—poisoning from a vitamin build-up within the body (see Table 1 for signs of Vitamin A toxicity). The information you need about vitamins and minerals can be found in Appendix A.

In addition to the material given in the tables, it is important to know that vitamins are both fat-soluble and water-soluble. The fat-soluble vitamins, A, D, E, and K, dissolve in fat, and any excesses are stored in the body. The water-soluble vitamins, B-complex and C, do not build up in the body but

TABLE 1　　　**Signs of Vitamin A Toxicity**

Serum vitamin A of 250–6600 I.U./100 ml.
Bone pain and fragility
Hydrocephalus and vomiting (infants and children)
Dry, fissured skin
Brittle nails
Hair loss (alopecia)
Gingivitis
Cheilosis
Anorexia
Irritability
Fatigue
Hepatomegaly and abnormal liver function
Ascites and portal hypertension

SOURCE: Marie V. Krause and Kathleen L. Mahan, *Food, Nutrition, and Diet Therapy* (New York: Macmillan Publishing Company, 1977), p. 154.

are regularly excreted in the urine. (Doctors have been known to say that Americans have the most expensive urine in the world.) You should take care not to overconsume vitamins, both for your health's sake and for the health of your pocketbook.

CARBOHYDRATES   Carbohydrates are the body's primary source of energy because their simple molecular structure allows them to be metabolized more rapidly than fats or proteins. Sometimes called "brainfood," carbohydrates provide us with quick energy, which is why they are sometimes said to give us an "instant high." The traditional belief that fish and celery are "brainfoods" is a myth. Only carbohydrates supply fuel in a form that the brain can use.[15]

During digestion all carbohydrates are eventually broken down into glucose.[16] Glucose provides the major source of energy for body cells. Some carbohydrates are stored in the liver and muscles in the form of glycogen (an animal starch), which is then available for rapid conversion into glucose when extra energy is needed.[17]

Carbohydrates also help our body make better use of protein. If our carbohydrate intake is very low, the body will draw on protein for energy. But protein is an inefficient energy source because it requires additional metabolism before it can be used for that purpose. Furthermore, the by-products of metabolized protein must be excreted by the kidneys. (Organic gardeners have been known to add urine to compost piles because it is the richest natural source of nitrogen.)

All carbohydrates are either sugars or more complex compounds such as starch, which is formed by long chains of glucose molecules strung together.[18] Contrary to common opinion, it is not the "pure" sugar or candy bar that gives us the quick energy needed for sports or muscular activity, but rather a starchy food such as doughnuts, pasta, pancakes, oatmeal, or bread. This is because all carbohydrates must go through a conversion process, simple or complex, before being absorbed for energy. The carbohydrate content of several common foods is shown in Figure 1.

Another interesting bit of information refutes the idea that all foods should be eaten raw: for digestion to be complete, starch must be cooked in moist heat. The body can digest raw starchy food, but not as completely as it can absorb cooked starchy food.

PROTEIN   Protein is important to the diet for the growth, maintenance, and repair of tissue; however, it is probably the most overemphasized nutrient, and as a rule Americans consume too much of it.[19] (Consider the popularity of steak dinners or barbequed beef, and the statement "I'm a meat and potatoes man.") Protein is important, but no more or less important than

FIGURE 1 Carbohydrate Content of Common Foods

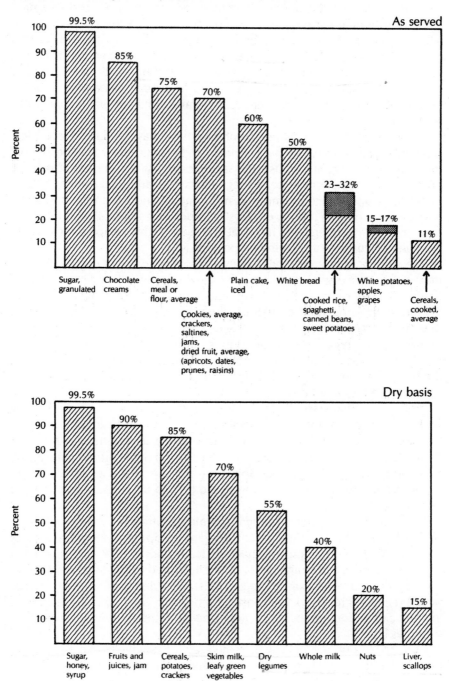

Source: George M. Briggs and Doris Howes Calloway, *Bogert's Nutrition and Physical Fitness* (Philadelphia: W. B. Saunders Company, 1979), p. 58.

other nutrients that make up a balanced diet.

Amino acids are the building blocks of protein, but the kind of amino acids vary in different proteins.[20] A protein containing the essential amino acids, which are those that cannot be manufactured in the body, is called a *complete protein*. Complete protein foods, generally animal or animal products, are meat, milk, eggs, cheese, poultry, and fish. Foods lacking one or more of the essential amino acids are said to contain *incomplete protein*. Examples of this type of protein are beans, grains, other vegetables and fruits, and, in general, plant foods.

When some plant foods are combined they may produce a complete protein. For example, whole wheat bread and peanut butter together supply the eight essential amino acids necessary to qualify as a complete protein, as do certain combinations of beans (legumes) with cornbread or rice. A complete discussion of the makeup of amino acids and their relationships is impossible to offer in a book of this size; strict vegetarians should therefore read one of the references listed at the end of this chapter for a more thorough discussion of protein composition.

The amount of protein needed daily by the average adult can be supplied in two four-ounce servings of meat plus two cups of milk.[21] However, lean tissue requires more protein for maintenance than fatty tissue requires. Therefore, growing children require more protein than adults; most males, due to a larger percentage of muscle, require more protein than most females; and a pregnant woman requires more protein than other women because she is supporting a developing child in addition to herself. Because the body does not store amino acids as such, it is important that protein be consumed on a daily basis.

Protein molecules are too large to be directly absorbed, so they must be broken down before they can be digested as a nutrient. Digestion begins in the stomach, but the major changes take place in the small intestine.[22] Protein digestion is more complex and takes longer than carbohydrate digestion, which is why protein-rich foods are not the best ones to eat before strenuous activity. (Marathon runners tend to load up on carbohydrates the day before a race.)

Protein is the only energy nutrient containing nitrogen. Protein molecules also contain carbon, hydrogen, and oxygen, as do the molecules of other nutrients.[23] When more protein than needed is consumed, the nitrogen will be removed from the amino acids by the liver and excreted in the form of urea by the kidney.[24] Excess protein puts a heavier load on the kidneys, which is another reason not to consume more than you need. The remaining amino acids become a source of quick energy; if they are not used they are stored as fat.

Contrary to popular beliefs, extremely active people do not need more protein than the average person, but all people need an adequate amount of protein throughout their lives—so it is not true that older people need less protein. As long as the body is producing new cells, which it must do to live, it needs adequate amounts of protein. The protein content of several common foods is shown in Figure 2.

To get a rough idea of your daily complete protein requirement (in grams), divide your body weight by 3;[25] grams can be converted to calories simply by multiplying by 4. (There are four calories in every gram of protein and carbohydrate, nine calories in every gram of fat.) A 144-pound person would need 8 grams (144 divided by 3) or 184 calories (46 × 4) of protein.

FIGURE 2   Protein Content of Some Typical Foods as Served

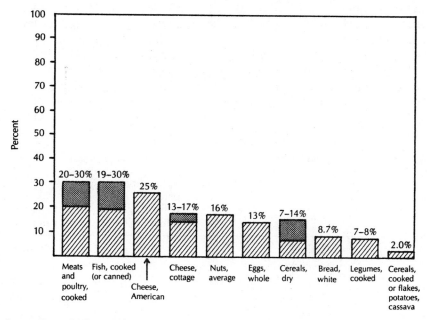

Source: George M. Briggs and Doris Howes Calloway, *Bogert's Nutrition and Physical Fitness* (Philadelphia: W. B. Saunders Company, 1979), p. 102.

FATS   Fats, also called *lipids,* are composed of carbon, hydrogen, and oxygen. They are different from carbohydrates because they contain less oxygen.[26] The core of the fat molecule is glycerol, with which three fatty acids combine to form the fat molecule.[27] This is why fat is also called a *tri*glyceride.

A pure triglyceride contains only identical fatty acids, whereas a triglyceride that contains different fatty acids is called a mixed triglyceride. Triglycerides, which are liquid at room temperature, are called *oils,* and those that are solid at room temperature are called *fats.*[28] As a rule, fats are more saturated and oils less saturated—or more *un*saturated (or polyunsaturated). (The degree of unsaturation is measured by iodine value; the relation between iodine value and unsaturation is shown in Table 2.) Generally, oils come from plants, and fats come from animals. A rule of thumb in determining the degree of saturation is to observe how hard a fat is at room temperature.[29] A harder fat is more saturated than a softer fat. A less saturated fat is considered more healthful.

Triglycerides comprise approximately 98 percent of the fats in foods and over 90 percent of the body's fat.[30] The remaining fat in food and in the body is made up of phospholipids and sterols (most importantly, cholesterol). Cholesterol is not necessarily as dangerous as many people think. Many other factors, such as obesity, lack of exercise, smoking, and hypertension, may be more important causes of increased cholesterol deposits in the arteries, which restrict arterial flexibility and may cause heart disease.

Fats are a concentrated form of energy, which means that only small amounts of them are needed. They make food more appetizing and, in addition, they carry the fat-soluble vitamins. Fat also carries an essential

TABLE 2 **Relationship of Iodine Values to Polyunsaturation**

Oil source	Approximate percent polyunsaturation	Iodine value
Safflower	78	140–150
Soybean	62	125–135
Corn oil	58	110–128
Cottonseed	54	100–115
Peanut	33	85–100
Lard	10	55–70
Palm	10	45–55
Butterfat	4	25–40
Cocoa butter	4	30–40
Palm kernel	2	15–25
Coconut oil	2	5–15

NOTE: Iodine value is a measure of the degree of unsaturation of a lipid.

SOURCE: P. L. White, D. C. Fletcher, and M. Ellis, eds., *Nutrients in Processed Foods: Fats and Carbohydrates* (Acton, Mass., Publishing Sciences Group, Inc., 1975), p. 18.

nutrient, linoleic acid. Dermatitis—a skin disease—is one of the results of a lack of this important nutrient in the diet.

Lipids also serve as a reserve source of energy.[31] However, too large a reserve of energy results in obesity. Lipids are found in fats and oils as well as in fish, poultry, beef, and pork. Fat is also found in milk and milk products, eggs, butter, many prepared and frozen foods, lunch meats, and so on. Eating these foods *in moderation* will not make the average person tend to put on fat. (Typical fat-rich foods are shown in Figure 3.)

The energy value of food is measured in units of heat, or calories. Food does not contain calories; rather it has energy potential measured in calories.[32] In order to determine the energy value of food, a sample is actually burned in a laboratory in a device called a calorimeter. This is how the calorie ratings of foods are determined.

Activity can also be measured in terms of calories. One pound of fat is equal to 3,500 calories. This information can be used to create an energy

FIGURE 3 Typical Fat-Rich Foods

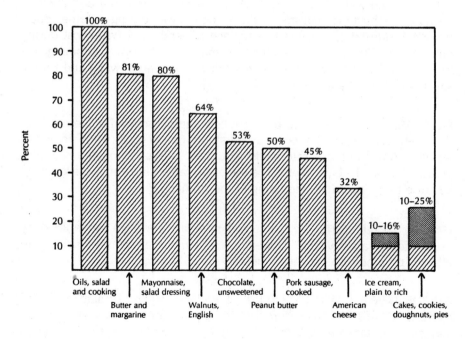

Source: George M. Briggs and Doris Howes Calloway, *Bogert's Nutrition and Physical Fitness* (Philadelphia: W. B. Saunders Company, 1979), p. 72.

balance between food intake and activity output in order to maintain a certain weight or to lose or gain weight. Simply, when more calories are consumed than are used in activity, there will be a gain in weight. Conversely, when fewer calories are consumed than are used in activity, weight will be lost. If there is a magic formula, this is it!

Health foods are not lower in calories; in fact, the best "health food" is found in the fresh meat, produce, vegetable, and fruit sections of the grocery store. Protein supplements and megadoses of vitamins are really unnecessary and quite expensive.

NUTRITION AND SPORTS

Current research has proven some past practices in athletic nutrition to be false and even dangerous. Coaches, athletes, and all persons, male or female, who engage in strenuous activity or voluntary competition must practice caution where breakthroughs in athletic nutrition are concerned.

WATER   Excessive water losses can cause mental confusion as well as severe discomfort during activity.[33] During competition an athlete should drink as much water as desired. However, even that may not be sufficient, because the thirst mechanism does not function well during extreme conditions.[34] Sports drinks are used to replace minerals and water lost during competition. This type of drink can be made at home by combining one third to one half a teaspoon of iodized salt with a quart of water and adding sugar and flavoring, if desired.[35]

SALT TABLETS   Most active people receive ample sodium in their normal diets, enough to sustain even a marathon runner competing in warm weather. Any additional salt needs should be satisfied through a slight increase of salt in the basic diet.[36] The use of salt tablets is strongly discouraged because they can irritate the lining of the stomach.[37]

VITAMIN SUPPLEMENTS   Vitamin and mineral needs are determined by body size, not activity level. Therefore, supplements are of no extra value to athletes on a normal, balanced diet.[38]

CARBOHYDRATE LOADING   During an endurance type of activity which exceeds forty-five minutes duration, the usual supply of stored energy is sometimes insufficient to supply the energy needed.[39] Research has shown that energy stores can be increased through a process called carbohydrate loading. The process usually involves a six-day period of time. On the first day, the athlete takes a long workout to completely exhaust the muscles used in competition. The next two days involve light activity or rest. During these three days, the diet consists primarily of protein and fats and is *very* low in carbohydrates. The athlete engages in a hard workout again on the fourth day while changing the diet to a high carbohydrate intake, low in protein and fats. The next two days before competition involve rest and a diet that is high in carbohydrates and low in protein and fats. On the day of competition, the diet consists of all carbohydrates or high carbohydrates. Sugar drinks are also added on the day of competition.

For most athletes, it is advisable to limit carbohydrate loading to important competitions.[40] Also, because there has been some concern voiced by physicians over possible side-effects, such as stiff and heavy-feeling muscles, carbohydrate loading should be practiced only under the supervision of knowledgeable personnel.[41]

THE PREGAME MEAL   Meals consumed before competition should be eaten no less than two hours before activity begins in order to ensure that the stomach and upper bowels are relatively empty. Carbohydrates are the most efficient foods since they are digested and metabolized more rapidly and do not have the dehydrating characteristic of proteins.[42] Competitors should stay with foods that are familiar to them. Also, they will be more comfortable if they consume less of the foods that have a tendency to cause gas, such as beans, cabbage, turnips, and certain other fruits and vegetables as well as some seasonings. Care should be taken to avoid foods that are highly salted, such as nuts, chips, or popcorn.[43] Whole milk should be eliminated from the pregame meal because of its high fat content. Caffeine drinks can cause an increase in tension and sometimes can cause a hypoglycemic reaction and must also be excluded. Caffeine drinks include not only coffee and tea but also colas.

Athletes should develop a constant awareness of their nutritional status because of its importance to health and its effect on competition. The most important consideration concerning the composition of meals prior to competition is that they should not interfere with the physical and psychological stresses that surround performance.[44]

ALCOHOL AND DRUGS   Unquestionably, these are not recommended. Tobacco smoking definitely hinders neuromuscular and cardiovascular performance. Alcohol is a depressant, metabolizes slowly, and dehydrates—all of which are detrimental to any type of activity. The practice of mixing alcohol, strong drugs, and strenuous exercise can actually be dangerous to the point of death.

WEIGHT LOSS DURING TRAINING   Most athletes need a minimum of 2,000 calories during training; in fact, 3,000 to 5,000 calories is not unusual. If severe weight-loss programs are attempted during this time, they would cause a reduction in muscle tissue rather than fat. Restricting water intake to induce weight loss, as wrestlers frequently do, can even be dangerous.[45] Weight-loss programs are best attempted during the off-season when the exercise is not as strenuous.

WEIGHT GAIN   Weight gain is accomplished by increasing the intake of calories through a balanced diet. Specific training and conditioning programs should accompany the high caloric intake, if muscle and not fat is to be the major tissue component of added weight.[46] Since exercise does not lead to a significant increase in the amount of protein metabolized, diets that call for a high intake of protein in order to build muscle mass have no real validity.[47] The maximum weight gain recommended is approximately two to three pounds per week.[48] Using anabolic steroids and hormones to induce weight gain is hazardous—they are of questionable value in improving performance, and there is no doubt that they contribute to diminished testicular function in males and can permanently damage reproductive tissues.[49]

It can be seen that if the energy intake exceeds the energy outgo, an individual is in positive energy balance. Since the law of the conservation of energy tells us that energy can neither be gained nor lost but only changed in form, we must look for this energy to be deposited in the form of body fat, which is indeed what happens.

—HERBERT deVRIES
Physiology of Exercise

CONCLUSION

The study of nutrition and foods is of most importance in controlling weight and maintaining health. All of us should be aware of the foods we are eating and the effect they have on the body. With a knowledge of basic nutritional principles, food intake can be controlled, even when most meals are eaten outside of the home. If we choose the correct foods, we can eat almost anywhere. Becoming knowledgeable and applying that knowledge is the key to success.

Notes

1. Arthur C. Guyton, *Textbook of Medical Physiology* (Philadelphia: W. B. Saunders Company, 1976), p. 63.
2. Ruth L. Carey, Irma B. Vyhmeister, and Jeannie S. Hudson, *Commonsense Nutrition* (Mountain View: Pacific Press Publishing Association, 1971), p. 14.
3. Corrinne H. Robinson, *Basic Nutrition and Diet Therapy*, 3rd ed. (New York: Macmillan Publishing Company, 1975), p. 4.
4. Fredrick J. Stare and Margaret McWilliams, *Living Nutrition* (New York: John Wiley and Sons, 1973), pp. 3–6.
5. Robinson, *Basic Nutrition*, p. 25.
6. *Ibid.*, p. 26.
7. Eva D. Wilson, Katherine H. Fisher, and Mary F. Fuqua, *Principles of Nutrition* (New York: John Wiley and Sons, Inc., 1975), p. 110.
8. Robinson, p. 26.
9. *Ibid.*
10. *Ibid.*, p. 44.
11. Wilson, Fisher, and Fuqua, *Principles of Nutrition*, p. 202.
12. Ronald M. Deutsch, *Realities of Nutrition* (Palo Alto: Bull Publishing Company, 1976), p. 227.
13. Marie V. Krause and Kathleen L. Mahan, *Food, Nutrition and Diet Therapy* (Philadelphia: W. B. Saunders Company, 1979), p. 185.
14. Corrinne H. Robinson and Marilyn R. Lawler, *Normal and Therapeutic Nutrition* (New York: Macmillan Publishing Company, 1977), p. 149.
15. George M. Briggs and Doris Howes Calloway, *Bogert's Nutrition and Physical Fitness* (Philadelphia: W. B. Saunders Company, 1979), p. 357.
16. Nathan J. Smith, *Food for Sport* (Palo Alto: Bull Publishing Company, 1976), p. 12.
17. Briggs and Calloway, *Bogert's Nutrition*, p. 358.
18. *Ibid.*, pp. 50–51.
19. Deutsch, *Realities of Nutrition*, p. 193.
20. Wilson, Fisher, and Fuqua, p. 67.
21. Stare and McWilliams, *Living Nutrition*, p. 291.
22. Wilson, Fisher, and Fuqua, p. 107.
23. Briggs and Calloway, p. 82.
24. Robinson, p. 45.
25. Deutsch, p. 196.
26. Robinson, p. 50.
27. Wilson, Fisher, and Fuqua, p. 51.
28. *Ibid.*
29. Guyton, *Textbook of Medical Physiology*, p. 6.
30. Robinson and Lawler, *Normal and Therapeutic Nutrition*, p. 77.
31. Deutsch, p. 38.
32. *Ibid.*, p. 41.
33. Ellington Darden, *Nutrition and Athletic Performance* (Pasadena: The Athletic Press, 1976), p. 121.

34. *Ibid.*, p. 116.
35. Darden, *Nutrition and Athletic Performance*, p. 125; Smith, *Food for Sport*, p. 97.
36. Smith, p. 97.
37. Darden, p. 159.
38. Darden, p. 45; Smith, p. 99.
39. Darden, p. 116.
40. Smith, p. 84.
41. Briggs and Calloway, p. 533.
42. Smith, p. 119.
43. *Ibid.*, p. 124.
44. Darden, p. 167.
45. *Ibid.*, p. 143.
46. Smith, p. 63.
47. Darden, p. 88.
48. Smith, p. 63.
49. *Ibid.*, p. 64.

4 | *WEIGHT CONTROL*

For many of us, overeating has become a way of life. Approximately one fifth of all adults in the United States are moderately overweight, and obesity has become one of our major health problems.[1] Weight control is an important component of physical fitness, one that will determine one's ability to achieve maximum fitness.

CAUSES AND RISKS OF OBESITY

CAUSES   When the food intake level exceeds the energy expenditure, the result will be a gain in weight. The excess food is stored as fat. Whatever the indirect cause, the direct cause is that the obese individual consumes more food than needed and usually does not engage in enough exercise.

Eating patterns, an indirect cause of obesity, are established early in life. Overfeeding during a child's early, formative years will plant the seed for future weight problems. Research points out that overfeeding during this stage can actually result in an increase in the size and number of fat cells within the body, making it more difficult to control weight as an adult.[2]

There are many more indirect causes of obesity: emotional overeating, illness or accident resulting in inactivity, sedentary living, and types of food consumed are some of them. Whatever the cause, the result is an uneven balance of energy output and intake.

RISKS   Obesity obviously affects appearance, but the physiological problems associated with carrying too much fat are not so obvious. The kidneys do not respond as well in disposing of fluids, which results in fluid retention making it more difficult to lose weight. The metabolizing of food becomes less efficient, and more of the nutrients are converted to fat for storage. Obese individuals are more susceptible to diseases such as diabetes, gall bladder problems, appendicitis, respiratory disorders, and heart disease.[3] In addition, obesity slows recovery from surgery, and in many instances, the mortality rate for obese individuals is higher.

FAD DIETS

Every month many popular magazines publish the latest fad diets, and others carry advertisements for highly questionable weight-control products.

The purported magical formulas for losing weight—such as the grapefruit and water diet, egg diets, all-protein diets, and so on—are effective only when they cause you to cut calories. In some instances, their concentration on one type of food, whether it be high in protein, carbohydrate, or fat, can lead to health problems. According to Dr. Neil Solomon: "fad diets tend to throw the metabolism out of balance and setting it straight again is difficult. When the individual begins eating normally again, he may store more fat than he would if his body were behaving properly."[4]

> *Weight control has become a matter of intense interest. Out of this concern for weight control has grown an industry, much of it impregnated with quackery, which produces sensational books, pills of various colors, and potencies, belts, weights, corsets, steam baths, and so on, which are peddled to a desperate and credulous clientele.*
>
> —JEAN MEYER
> *Health*

It should be obvious that fad diets, no matter how attractive they may seem, are nutritionally unbalanced and cannot be used as a long-term answer to weight control.

Any good weight-control program must meet two criteria: (1) the development of a lifetime balanced diet plan, and (2) the regulation of caloric intake and output. The remainder of this chapter concentrates on ways in which you can develop a personal program that meets these two criteria.

DEVELOPING A BALANCED DIET

When the intake of calories is reduced, there is a corresponding decrease in the amount of vitamins and minerals consumed. To compensate for this, extra care must be taken when making food choices.

U.S. RECOMMENDED DAILY ALLOWANCE (U.S. RDA)   The U.S. Recommended Daily Allowance (U.S. RDA) chart, independently researched and published by the United States government, gives the daily requirements for many vitamins and common minerals. Use of this chart will ensure that normal vitamin and mineral needs are being met. A recent U.S. RDA chart is shown in Table 3.

As an aid to consumers, most food manufacturers are including U.S. RDA percentages on their nutritionally labeled foods. An example is shown in Table 4. Make it a habit to buy products with high U.S. RDA percentages.

THE BASIC FOUR FOOD GROUPS   The variety of foods available can make selecting a U.S. RDA balanced diet very time-consuming. However, the Basic Four Chart (Figure 4) provides a reliable shortcut toward achieving dietary balance. Serving sizes for the basic four food groups are listed below.

Milk and cheese	Milk: 1 cup, 8 oz Cheese: 1 slice, 1" × 1" × 2" slice Cottage cheese: 1¼ cup Ice cream: 1¼ cup
Meat	Lean meat: 2–3 oz Poultry, fish: 2–3 oz Eggs: 2 Cooked beans or peas: 1 cup Peanut butter: 4 tsp
Vegetables and fruits	½ cup or whole piece
Cereal	Bread: 1 slice Cereal: 1 oz Cooked cereal: ½–¾ cup Macaroni, rice: ½–¾ cup Noodles, spaghetti: ½–¾ cup

It is important that you distribute servings from each group throughout the day in order to maximize nutritional value.

TABLE 3 U.S. Recommended Daily Dietary Allowances (Revised 1979)

	Age (years)	Weight (kg)	Weight (lb)	Height (cm)	Height (in)	Protein (g)	Fat-Soluble Vitamins Vitamin A (µg R.E.)ᵃ	Vitamin D (µg)ᵇ	Vitamin E (mg α T.E.)ᶜ	Water-Soluble Vitamins Vitamin C (mg)	Thiamin (mg)	Riboflavin (mg)	Niacin (mg N.E.)ᵈ	Vitamin B6 (mg)	Folacinᵉ (µg)	Vitamin B12 (µg)	Minerals Calcium (mg)	Phosphorus (mg)	Magnesium (mg)	Iron (mg)	Zinc (mg)	Iodine (µg)
Infants	0.0–0.5	6	13	60	24	kg × 2.2	420	10	3	35	0.3	0.4	6	0.3	30	0.5ᶠ	360	240	50	10	3	40
	0.5–1.0	9	20	71	28	kg × 2.0	400	10	4	35	0.5	0.6	8	0.6	45	1.5	540	360	70	15	5	50
Children	1–3	13	29	90	35	23	400	10	5	45	0.7	0.8	9	0.9	100	2.0	800	800	150	15	10	70
	4–6	20	44	112	44	30	500	10	6	45	0.9	1.0	11	1.3	200	2.5	800	800	200	10	10	90
	7–10	28	62	132	52	34	700	10	7	45	1.2	1.4	16	1.6	300	3.0	800	800	250	10	10	120
Males	11–14	45	99	157	62	45	1000	10	8	50	1.4	1.6	18	1.8	400	3.0	1200	1200	350	18	15	150
	15–18	66	145	176	69	56	1000	10	10	60	1.4	1.7	18	2.0	400	3.0	1200	1200	400	18	15	150
	19–22	70	154	177	70	56	1000	7.5	10	60	1.5	1.7	19	2.2	400	3.0	800	800	350	10	15	150
	23–50	70	154	178	70	56	1000	5	10	60	1.4	1.6	18	2.2	400	3.0	800	800	350	10	15	150
	51+	70	154	178	70	56	1000	5	10	60	1.2	1.4	16	2.2	400	3.0	800	800	350	10	15	150
Females	11–14	46	101	157	62	46	800	10	8	50	1.1	1.3	15	1.8	400	3.0	1200	1200	300	18	15	150
	15–18	55	120	163	64	46	800	10	8	60	1.1	1.3	14	2.0	400	3.0	1200	1200	300	18	15	150
	19–22	55	120	163	64	44	800	7.5	8	60	1.1	1.3	14	2.0	400	3.0	800	800	300	18	15	150
	23–50	55	120	163	64	44	800	5	8	60	1.0	1.2	13	2.0	400	3.0	800	800	300	18	15	150
	51+	55	120	163	64	44	800	5	8	60	1.0	1.2	13	2.0	400	3.0	800	800	300	10	15	150
Pregnant						+30	+200	+5	+2	+20	+0.4	+0.3	+2	+0.6	+400	+1.0	+400	+400	+150	g	+5	+25
Lactating						+20	+400	+5	+3	+40	+0.5	+0.5	+5	+0.5	+100	+1.0	+400	+400	+150	g	+10	+50

SOURCE: Adapted from *Recommended Dietary Allowances*, Ninth Edition (1979, in press), with the permission of the National Academy of Sciences, Washington, D.C.

NOTE: The allowances are intended to provide for individual variations among most normal persons as they live in the United States under usual environmental stresses. Diets should be based on a variety of common foods in order to provide other nutrients for which human requirements have been less well defined.

ᵃRetinol equivalents. 1 Retinol equivalent = 1 µg retinol or 6 µg β-carotene.

ᵇAs cholecalciferol. 10 µg cholecalciferol = 400 I.U. vitamin D.

ᶜα-tocopherol equivalents. 1 mg d-α-tocopherol = 1 α T.E.

ᵈ1 NE (niacin equivalent) is equal to 1 mg of niacin or 60 mg of dietary tryptophan.

ᵉThe folacin allowances refer to dietary sources as determined by *Lactobacillus casei*

assay after treatment with enzymes ("conjugases") to make polyglutamyl forms of the vitamin available to the test organism.

ᶠThe RDA for vitamin B12 in infants is based on average concentration of the vitamin in human milk. The allowances after weaning are based on energy intake (as recommended by the American Academy of Pediatrics) and consideration of other factors such as intestinal absorption.

ᵍThe increased requirement during pregnancy cannot be met by the iron content of habitual American diets nor by the existing iron stores of many women; therefore the use of 30 – 60 mg of supplemental iron is recommended. Iron needs during lactation are not substantially different from those of nonpregnant women, but continued supplementation of the mother for 2 to 3 months after parturition is advisable in order to replenish stores depleted by pregnancy.

FIGURE 4
Four Food Groups-
A Daily Food Guide

MILK, CHEESE 2 or more servings (more for children)	MEAT, FISH, EGGS 2 or more servings
VEGETABLES, FRUITS 4 or more servings	BREAD, CEREALS 4 or more servings

and other foods as needed for complete and satisfying meals

Corinne Robinson, *Basic Nutrition and Diet Therapy*, 3rd ed. (New York: Macmillan Publishing Company, 1975), p. 35.

TABLE 4   **Nutrition Information**

(Per serving)
Serving size = 8 oz
Servings per container = 1

Calories	560
Protein	23 grams
Carbohydrate	43 grams
Fat (Percent of calories 53%)	33 grams
Polyunsaturated*	2 grams
Saturated	9 grams
Cholesterol* (20 mg/100 g)	40 milligrams
Sodium (365 mg/100 g)	830 milligrams

Percentage of U.S. recommended daily allowances (U.S. RDA)

Protein	35
Vitamin A	35
Vitamin C (ascorbic acid)	10
Thiamine (Vitamin B)	15
Riboflavin	15
Niacin	25
Calcium	2
Iron	25

*Information on fat and cholesterol content is provided for individuals who, on the advice of a physician, are modifying their total dietary intake of fat and cholesterol.
SOURCE: Corinne Robinson, *Basic Nutrition and Diet Therapy*, 3rd ed. (New York: Macmillan Publishing Company, 1975), p. 177.

REGULATING CALORIC INTAKE

Energy intake and output is measured in terms of calories. Whether the objective is to lose or to gain weight, you must have a knowledge of the caloric value of food. After that, it's just a matter of addition or subtraction.

Every stored pound of body fat represents an excess intake of 3,500 calories of food energy. If the daily caloric intake is decreased by 800 calories, the weight loss will be approximately 1.5 pounds a week. If the diet is increased by the same number of calories, the result will be just the opposite, a weight gain of 1.5 pounds a week.

It sounds simple, and it would be if we were totally physical beings and did not have minds or feelings to consider. It's easy to work the calculator—to add or subtract the calories and devise the menus—but that is only the beginning. The secret is in the application. In most cases, our pattern of living must be changed in order to achieve the results we want.

CHANGING HABIT PATTERNS

At the present time, the most successful method of changing habit patterns seems to be behavior modification. Its techniques can be used to change any unwanted habit; however, as you study this section, evaluate your behavior in relation to food. If you try, behavior modification can work for you!

One of the ironies of human health is that people often feel most helpless when they are least helpless. Individuals may have little control over the spread of disease germs through the environment, but they have a great deal of control over their own behavior. No one has more power than you have to determine whether you drink too much or smoke tobacco or overeat.

—INSEL and ROTH
Health in a Changing Society

STAGE ONE: COLLECT DATA Studies have shown that even calorie-conscious persons can be very inaccurate in their judgment of caloric intake. The best way of knowing conclusively is to keep exact records. Design a recording method to fit your own needs, then take the time to be an accurate record keeper. An example of one method is shown in Figure 5.

STAGE TWO: SPECIFY THE GENERAL PROBLEM AREA Are the foods you eat too rich in calories, or are your servings too large? Are the excessive

FIGURE 5   A Record of Food Intake

Calorie intake			Relevant information		
Food	Quan-tity	Calories	Time	Location	Circumstances
COFFEE SUGAR	1C 1t	0 16	8:15	KITCHEN	BREAKFAST — IN A HURRY
COFFEE SUGAR	1C 1t	0 16	10:15	WORK	COFFEE BREAK
SWEET ROLL	1	150			
CHEESE SANDWICH	1	285	12:15	RESTAURANT	LUNCH HOUR
SALAD WITH DRESSING	3C 2T	152			
COKE	8 oz.	100			
ICE CREAM	8 oz.	300			
COKE	8 oz.	100	3:05	WORK	COFFEE BREAK
DONUT RAISED, JELLY	1	226			
CHEESE	2"x2" x3"	125	5:30	KITCHEN	FIXING DINNER
SALAD WITH DRESSING	2C 3T	228	6:05	DINING ROOM	DINNER
BREAD	2 SLICES	124			
STEAK	4 oz.	260			
CAKE CHOC. W/ ICING	1/8 TH	350	8:45	DEN	WATCHING T.V.
COKE	12 oz. CAN	150	9:30	DEN	WATCHING T.V.

calories confined to a few problem foods—such as candy or colas? Do you drink too many high-calorie alcoholic drinks before dinner? Do you exercise regularly?

STAGE THREE: IDENTIFY PATTERNS   At what time do you eat the most empty calories? Are you watching television when this occurs? Do you snack immediately before a large meal? Are your food snacks just a hand or step away from where you sit? Consider all factors related to your eating habits.

STAGE FOUR: EXAMINE POSSIBLE SOLUTIONS   In what ways can you change your behavior, locations, or timing? Try to be innovative and imaginative in your thinking. Once you have chosen some solutions, imagine yourself practicing those actions. This may be a help in anticipating problems.

STAGE FIVE: NARROW THE OPTIONS AND EXPERIMENT   Examine your solutions, keeping in mind what you could *realistically* accept as a change in your lifestyle. (Do not decide to jog every night if you dislike running!) From those options remaining, pick the one that offers the best possibility for success.

STAGE SIX: COMPARE CURRENT AND PAST DATA   Do not expect total success immediately. Accept the fact that you have practiced certain behavior patterns for a long time. It takes time to change—one or two weeks is not long enough.

STAGE SEVEN: EXTEND, REVISE, OR REPLACE SOLUTIONS   You can learn from your errors! Be prepared to change or refine your solution if it was unsuccessful. If your solution did work, try to find ways to reinforce your successful strategy.[5]

Behavior modification specialists believe that what you think in your head is more important than what you feel in your stomach. You must learn to let your thinking work *for* you instead of *against* you.[6] They also recommend allowing some leeway in changing behavior. Committing yourself to an "always" or "never again" goal does not allow for the occasional backsliding that usually accompanies gradual change.[7]

Farmers who want fat hogs, geese, and steers keep them penned up and eating. Trainers of race horses and managers of boxers rely on a combination of rationing and exercise to keep their charges trim.

FREMES and SABRY
Nutriscore

EXERCISE AND WEIGHT CONTROL

The effect of exercise on weight control is not to be discounted. Regular exercise increases the activity level, which in turn causes the individual to use more calories. Table 5 will give you an idea of the amount of activity it takes to burn up the calories in certain foods.

During exercise a mechanism in the brain called the *appestat* adjusts feelings of hunger to activity level, causing a slight increase in appetite. However, as the level of activity increases, this effect begins to level off until, at high levels of exertion, there is actually a decrease in appetite. Conversely, at the sedentary level the appestat does not work well either. This explains why many obese people cannot recognize when their feelings of hunger have been satisfied.[8]

TABLE 5   **Expenditure of Calories for Various Activities**

Consider only the time spent in actual activity. Multiply your body weight by the number of calories given for each activity. The result will show the calories you use per minute. Remember that the figures given are averages and results will differ slightly even for individuals of identical body weight.

Type of activity	Calories used per lb per min
Sleeping	0.008
Sitting or eating	0.010
Typing (electric)	0.012
Typing (manual)	0.014
Driving a car	0.015
Standing	0.016
Bathing or dressing	0.017
Cooking or meal preparation	0.021
Painting (house)	0.023
Walking (2 mph)	0.023
Cleaning (house)	0.025
Baseball or softball	0.031
Dancing (slow)	0.031
Bicycling (5.5 mph)	0.033
Fencing (moderate)	0.033
Football (moderate)	0.033
Archery	0.034
Golf (twosome)	0.036
Badminton (moderate)	0.037

Table 5 continued

Type of activity	Calories used per lb per min
Volleyball (moderate)	0.037
Swimming (2.5 mph)	0.040
Boxing (nonstop)	0.044
Walking (downstairs)	0.044
Walking (4.5 mph)	0.044
Basketball (moderate)	0.046
Table tennis	0.046
Dancing (vigorous)	0.046
Horseback riding (trot)	0.046
Tennis (moderate)	0.046
Waterskiing	0.052
Weight training	0.052
Soccer (moderate)	0.060
Gardening (nonstop/vigorous)	0.062
Handball	0.065
Racquetball	0.066
Skating (vigorous)	0.068
Squash	0.069
Mountain climbing	0.070
Bicycling (13 mph)	0.071
Jogging (5.5 mph)	0.071
Skiing (5 mph)	0.077
Calisthenics (nonstop/vigorous)	0.097
Running (9 mph)	0.103
Walking (upstairs)	0.116
Stationary running (140 counts per min)	0.162

SOURCES: J.V.G.A. Durnin and R. Passmore, *Energy, Work and Leisure* (London: Heineman Educational Books, Ltd., 1967), pp. 49–76; C. F. Consolazio, R. R. Johnson, and I. J. Pecora, *Physiological Measurements of Metabolic Functions in Man* (New York: McGraw-Hill, 1963), pp. 330–32; Clara Mae Taylor, *Food Values in Shares and Weights* (New York: Macmillan Publishing Company, 1959), p. 12; and Phillip E. Allesen, Joyce M. Harrison, and Barbara Vance, *Fitness for Life* (Dubuque: W. C. Brown Company Publishers, 1976), pp. 89–96.

Table 6 sources

SOURCES: Linda Garrison, Phyllis Leslie, and Deborah Blackmore, *Fitness and Figure Control: The Creation of You* (Palo Alto: Mayfield Publishing Company, 1974), p. 95; U. S. Department of Agriculture, Publication 547, Washington D.C. (1969), p. 7; *Recommended Dietary Allowances*, Food and Nutrition Board, National Academy of Sciences, National Research Council (1979, in press); M. L. Hathaway and E. D. Foard, *Heights and Weights of Adults in the United States*, Home Economics Research Report No. 10, U. S. Department of Agriculture (Washington D.C.), Table 80, p. 111.

TABLE 6   Ideal Weight Chart

A weight chart should be used as a guide only. Individuals differ according to heredity, racial characteristics, bone or frame size, and amount of muscular and fatty tissue. Your basic bone structure and amount of muscular tissue determine whether you fall toward the lean or heavy end of the weight range for your height. Muscular tissue will be greater if you engage in activity that requires heavy lifting, such as weight lifting, ballet (which requires lifting your weight), or work on a road crew or at a shipping dock. Remember that muscle weighs more than fat but consumes less space. The most important thing is how you look in the mirror. If you are happy with your body build or figure, then don't worry about it!

Always weigh in the nude and measure your height without shoes. Compare your weight only on the same set of scales because scales can differ by as much as five pounds.

Weight range for men (pounds)	Height	Weight range for women (pounds)
	4'10"	87–105
	4'11"	91–109
105–130	5'0"	95–113
109–134	5'1"	99–117
112–138	5'2"	103–121
115–141	5'3"	107–125
119–145	5'4"	111–129
122–149	5'5"	115–133
126–153	5'6"	119–137
130–158	5'7"	123–141
134–163	5'8"	127–145
138–168	5'9"	131–149
142–173	5'10"	135–154
146–177	5'11"	139–159
150–181	6'0"	143–163
154–184	6'1"	147–167
158–189	6'2"	151–171
162–194	6'3"	
166–199	6'4"	
170–203	6'5"	
175–209	6'6"	
179–214	6'7"	
184–220	6'8"	

TIPS

WEIGH EVERY DAY   We can normally expect a small fluctuation from our ideal weight (see Table 6). However, when this amounts to a gain of three to four pounds, it is time to act! By now we should realize that it is much easier to keep weight off than to lose it once it has become a permanent part of our body.

LOSE WEIGHT SLOWLY   Weight accumulation is a relatively slow process, and too rapid a loss can cause a strain on the systems of the body to readjust. A loss of more than two pounds a week could also mean a loss of muscle tissue.[9]

EAT A GOOD BREAKFAST   In the morning the body is recovering from a 10 to 12 hour fast and needs fuel. Studies have proved that skipping breakfast impairs mid-morning efficiency as well as possibly causing an abnormal increase in appetite later in the day.[10] Breakfast should provide approximately 25 percent of your daily calories and should contain at least one food from each of the basic four food groups.[11]

EAT SLOWLY   Food is metabolized at a much slower rate than it is eaten. It takes about 20 to 30 minutes for the more quickly digested carbohydrates to enter the blood stream and notify the appestat that the body has been fed.[12] Most of us can easily eat past the point of fullness in that time.

Apply behavior modification techniques to your eating habits—for example, concentrate on chewing slowly, enjoying each unique taste; lay your fork or spoon down between bites; and use smaller dishes.

CONCLUSION

Lifetime weight control is possible only when the desire to lose weight becomes more important than the momentary pleasure of indulgence. The decision is yours. You really can lose weight if you want to!

Notes
1. Ruth L. Carey, Irma B. Vyhmeister, and Jeannie S. Hudson, *Commonsense Nutrition* (Mountain View: Pacific Press Publishing Association, 1971), p. 103.
2. Ronald M. Deutsch, *The Family Guide to Better Food and Better Health* (Des Moines: The Meredith Corporation, 1971), p. 109.
3. Fredrick J. Stare and Margaret McWilliams, *Living Nutrition* (New York: John Wiley and Sons, Inc., 1973), p. 93.

4. Neil Solomon and Sally Sheppard, *The Truth about Weight Control* (New York: Setin and Day, Inc., 1971), p. 93.

5. Michael J. Mahoney and Kathryn Mahoney, *Permanent Weight Control* (New York: W. W. Norton & Company, Inc., 1976), pp. 32–37.

6. *Ibid.,* p. 48.

7. *Ibid.,* p. 51.

8. Deutsch, *Family Guide to Better Food and Better Health,* p. 121.

9. Ellington Darden, *Nutrition and Athletic Performance* (Pasadena: The Athletic Press, 1976), p. 381.

10. Corrinne H. Robinson and Marilyn R. Lawler, *Normal and Therapeutic Nutrition* (New York: Macmillan Publishing Company, 1977), p. 209.

11. Darden, *Nutrition and Athletic Performance.*

12. Deutsch, p. 151.

5 | *BEGINNING AN EXERCISE PROGRAM*

Few Americans participate regularly in a planned program of physical activity, a program designed to improve their level of physical fitness. Some may be unconcerned; some may care but be ignorant of how to achieve their goals. Motivation is enhanced by success. If we have tried to design an exercise program around the wrong principles, we have probably become disenchanted. This chapter looks at physical fitness— what it is and how it can be improved, the correct principles of exercise, the relationship of posture to exercise, and the effects of stress on fitness.

PHYSICAL FITNESS

Physical fitness is a combination of three different but very important components, which are discussed in detail in Chapters 6, 7, and 8: endurance, flexibility, and strength. Although important for different reasons, each of the three plays an important role in creating the physically fit individual.

Cardiovascular and respiratory endurance is the ability to continue work or activity for long periods of time. This type of endurance is primarily concerned with the heart, lungs, and circulatory and respiratory systems, and it is developed through vigorous and prolonged exercise.

Flexibility is the range of movement of which the joints of the body are capable. The degree of flexibility possessed varies with each joint. Flexibility is developed through the use of slow, stretching exercises. The terms *power* and *agility* are sometimes referred to as components of physical fitness. We consider these factors to be encompassed by strength and flexibility, respectively.

Strength is the ability to exert muscular force. It is an important consideration in the performance of everyday activities, and it is improved by the use
of exercises that require lifting or pushing weights or objects.

The term total fitness incorporates the emotional, mental, and spiritual
aspects of fitness, as well as the physical. Although all these aspects are
important, in this book we deal specifically with the physical aspects of
fitness.

> *Even a person whose capacity is severely limited, either as a
> result of injury or due to a congenital defect, may develop
> the body so that it functions at its maximal level. What is
> important is that each individual plan a program that will
> keep the body working at top capacity and efficiency.*
>
> —JOHN LA PLACE
> *Health*

THE PRINCIPLES OF CONDITIONING

Certain factors must be present in order for exercise to be successful. This
section presents the principles of successful conditioning.

THE OVERLOAD PRINCIPLE   To improve any physical function, it is necessary to place that function under a repeatedly greater than normal work load
until it has adapted to the increased demands.[1] Overload, simply, means
doing more tomorrow than you did today. In order to become more physically fit, you must perform more activity than your body is accustomed to.
The degree of improvement is directly proportional to the intensity of the
overload.[2] The four basic methods of applying the overload principle are:

1. Increase the amount of resistance by adding more weight, increasing the
   force, or adjusting to the pull of gravity by changing body positions.
2. Increase the amount of work by adding to the number of repetitions, or
   by using exercises in succession for each part of the body.
3. Alter the duration of the work by holding a position longer, or by doing
   an equal amount of work in a shorter period of time.
4. Adjust the rest periods by decreasing the time between exercises.

Table 7 describes how to apply the overload principle to endurance,
flexibility, and strength exercises.

TABLE 7   Applications of the Overload Principle

Overload	Endurance	Flexibility	Strength
Resistance		Change body positions	Add additional weight or load
Workload	Increase distance covered	Add additional exercises	Increase number of repetitions
Duration	Decrease time taken to do same work or activity, or increase time and add more work	Hold exercise positions for longer period of time	Hold muscle contractions for longer period of time or decrease the time it takes to do the same work
Rest periods	Decrease or shorten rest periods or increase time between rest periods		Decrease or shorten rest periods or increase time between rest periods

THE **SAID** PRINCIPLE   This is a unifying principle that applies to any of the characteristics that comprise physical fitness.[3] SAID, Specific Adaptations to Imposed Demands, means simply that the human body will adapt specifically to exercise or activity. In order to obtain results from an exercise program, the demands must be sufficient to force adaptation.[4] This principle also applies in reverse, because the body will adapt specifically to inactivity as well. Both exercise and inactivity will cause our bodies to develop a certain posture, though it is probably the posture of the active person that we admire.

Knowledge of both the overload principle and the SAID principle can be helpful in setting up an exercise program. In order to achieve the greatest benefits from an exercise program, the demands of that program must be increased on a regular basis by using the overload principle.

WARM UP

Before beginning any specific exercise program, it is most important to allow time for the body to shift from the resting state to the moving or active state. The most effective warm-up is one that gradually works into the exercise program. The warm-up activity should relate specifically to the type of exercise program. For instance, light jogging relates to endurance exercise; light stretching, to flexibility exercise; and light lifting, to strength exercise.

The warm-up should result in an increase of the heart rate as well as an increase in the temperature of the muscles. It has also been shown that maximal oxygen intake is slightly higher after warming up, which would seem to indicate an improvement in efficiency.[5]

Most authorities believe that warming up before athletic competition helps prevent injury, and tests have shown that warming up before exercise can definitely prevent much of the muscle soreness that comes from first attempts at an exercise program.

> In an average high school of two thousand students, it is now easy for eighteen hundred to graduate without ever having contemplated the health problems they will be living with for the next half-century, and there is little chance that they will become familiar with exercise programs that would enable them to live longer and operate more effectively.
>
> —JAMES A. MICHENER
> *Sport in America*

Mental preparation is an important part of any warm-up program. If you have a negative attitude toward exercise, you will find it very difficult to really "get into" your exercise program. This aspect of your warm-up will take more time and will be more difficult on some days than on others. Sometimes you just will not feel like exercising. You are probably experiencing an emotional low. During these times, spend more time in your physical warm-up, change your music or turn it up so that it is louder, and make certain your music is happy and vigorous. Try to take your mind off the events of the day and your feelings and throw yourself into the exercise. You may be amazed at the change in your outlook afterwards.

COOL DOWN

You must prepare your body for rest, just as you must prepare it for action. The cooling-down process allows time for the body systems to return to normal and aids in preventing a possible pooling of blood in the lower extremities, which is especially prevalent during endurance exercise. It also allows for the metabolic processes to return to the resting state.

Activity for cooling down is in many cases just a tapering off or a slowing down of your exercise program, and gradually coming to a stop instead of ending abruptly. For instance, in an endurance program, slow your running to a jogging movement, then gradually taper off to a fast walk, and then a slower walk. In addition, endurance and strength exercise programs should be followed by a short period of slow stretching. Use the exercises described in Chapter 7 and stretch each major joint area.

> *While a warm-up is a generally accepted practice, few people realize that the body also needs a cooling-down period after exercise. They slump into complete relaxation immediately after exercise. This can cause dizzy spells, fainting and even more serious consequences. Strange as it seems, you must get ready for rest.*
>
> —KENNETH H. COOPER
> *The New Aerobics*

This information can be applied to living habits also. Apply the cool-down principles to relaxing before going to bed. Much of the insomnia that we experience might be alleviated if we gradually eased our minds and bodies into a sleeping posture. Instead, we expect to go directly into sleep from a tense, troubled, and in some cases, active posture. Try reading, listening to quiet music, television, or just meditating before retiring. These activities help place your mind and body in a sleeping mood.

THE STAGES OF EXERCISE

Our body adapts to exercise in steps or stages, just as the seasons allow us to adapt gradually to environmental changes. The exercise programs outlined in Chapters 6, 7, and 8 have been divided into three stages, allowing for a gradual adaptation of the body to the overload principle. The following general description will give you an idea of what to expect during each stage. The duration of each stage varies according to the type of exercise.

STAGE ONE: INITIATION   Stage One is a one- to three-week period of toughening up, in which a person unused to exercise will sometimes experience soreness as the waste products from exercise accumulate more quickly than the circulatory system can remove them.[6] The amount of discomfort varies depending upon the level of prior conditioning and the length of time the person has been inactive. Much of the soreness can be avoided by following the principles outlined earlier, and by easing gradually into the exercise program.

STAGE TWO: IMPROVEMENT   Stage Two lasts from six to ten weeks, and can be called the improvement stage, for it is during this time that a more obvious response is seen to the application of the overload principle.[7] Even though improvement is very obvious during this stage, you will still probably reach a plateau during this time during which improvement is minimal. You should expect this and accept it. Patience, persistence, and a gradual increase in the overload is necessary to overcome this seemingly static period.

STAGE THREE: MAINTENANCE   Stage Three lasts "forever." or for as long as you wish to maintain your level of physical fitness. This is appropriately called the maintenance stage. When a satisfactory level of physical fitness has been reached, overload is no longer necessary, and the workout sequence can be decreased to a minimum of three days per week if desired.[8]

EXERCISE SEQUENCE AND FREQUENCY

Workouts should be sufficiently spaced to allow for tissue growth and nutritional replenishment to take place, but with sufficient frequency to provide for physiological development.[9] Ideally, flexibility exercises should be performed daily, endurance work every other day, and heavy strength exercises three days a week. Better results will be obtained by exercising four to seven days a week than by doing all exercise programs in one or two long sessions a week.[10] In fact, some experts believe that only one exercise session a week can be more detrimental to the body than no exercise at all.[11]

The sequence we suggest for the different types of exercise is endurance, flexibility, and strength, in that order. Warm-up of a stretching nature should precede and follow any vigorous strength exercise program in order to prevent extreme muscle soreness. Endurance work is an excellent warm-up for a flexibility workout.

A MEDICAL EXAMINATION

A complete medical examination prior to beginning any exercise program is a necessity for anyone over the age of thirty. The examination should include both a resting and a stress electrocardiogram, and it should be repeated annually unless a pathological history indicates otherwise.

EXERCISE TIPS

Each exercise chapter contains general directions and a section of suggestions for making exercise easier and more enjoyable. The following suggestions are more general and apply to all types of exercise.

What time of day to exercise is a common question and a few myths exist in this area. Individual preference should be the criteria for choosing the time to exercise. Some persons function better early in the morning, whereas others can hardly muster the energy to go outside for the morning paper but are loaded with energy and ready for action once evening comes. Many business persons exercise during the lunch break. One thing is certain—you should not exercise immediately before or after a meal. This could disturb the digestive process. We suggest refraining from vigorous exercise for an hour before and two hours after each meal.

A degree of fatigue from exercising is to be expected, especially in the beginning. Rest periods during your exercising can help alleviate this condition when it occurs.[12] If your fatigue is severe and lasts for more than two hours after exercising, it is probably a sign that your exercise program has been too strenuous for your level of conditioning. If this is the case, you should reduce your workload. Other conditions can sometimes cause the fatigue factor to be extremely high; these include recovery from illness, illness itself, emotional tension and stress, or fear and anger. Do not discount these factors when evaluating your exercise program.

POSTURE

The physiological results of poor posture can have a lifelong effect. Body alignment even affects our psychological states. Since correct posture makes us look better, it improves our self-image and confidence.

The antigravity muscles, which are responsible for posture, work in pairs. When one side becomes weakened or inflexible, a deviation can result. For instance, weakened muscles in the upper back and neck can pull the head out of alignment; overdeveloped pectoral (chest) muscles can cause rounded shoulders, and weak abdominal muscles can lead to lower back pain.

If all body segments are balanced, an imaginary line will extend from the ear through the center of the shoulder to the center of the hip, behind the kneecap to the front of the ankle. Check your own alignment by having a friend hold a weighted string along the side of your body.

Most postural problems can be corrected or at least contained by strengthening the weakened antigravity muscles and following a flexibility exercise program. Use the exercises found in Chapters 7 and 8.

STRESS AND RELAXATION

Stressful situations are difficult if not impossible to avoid. Stress is a natural outcome of the pressures of living, and often results in a kind of body tension known as headache, backache, and eye-tic, and other disorders such as nausea and diarrhea. Since stress is inevitable, the problem becomes more a matter of learning how to cope with it rather than trying to avoid it.

> Conditioning by the moderate stress of a reasonable program of physical exercise sets up a cross resistance to various forms of pathogenic stress. By exercising intelligently a man can train his heart to resist attacks that might otherwise kill him. It doesn't matter if he has been training with calisthenics and is later attacked not by physical but by emotional stress. Cross resistance will help his heart stand off the attack in any case.
>
> —HERBERT deVRIES
> *Physiology of Exercise*

The ability to relax must become a part of your overall fitness program. The scope of this book does not permit a comprehensive discussion of the different methods of relaxation, but here are three that you can try:

1. Find a quiet place and lie down on the floor. Consciously relax all of the parts of your body. Start with your feet and work up the legs, through the trunk, to the arms, neck, and finally all parts of the face and head. Tell yourself to relax each part as you get to it.

2. If stress occurs as you are driving, find a place to stop the car. Grip the steering wheel as tightly as you can and hold for a count of ten. Then relax your grip and lean your head over onto the steering wheel and completely let go for a few minutes.

3. Practice this one anywhere. Close your eyes and think of a favorite retreat. Visualize the setting; hear the sounds; feel the air and smell the familiar smells. Let your mind go there for awhile.

You should remember that exercise alone will increase your ability to withstand all kinds of stress. As you become stronger physically, your emotional strength will increase as well. You will find that your ability to face stressful situations will improve.

CONCLUSION

Before beginning any exercise program, it is important to have a complete physical exam, especially if you are over thirty years old. The exam should include some type of stress testing where the heart is monitored during exercise. Then proceed with your exercise program as the doctor prescribes.

*Although one might expect that the human body will
eventually learn to react and to respond to the many stresses
of the present and future life as well as it learned to cope
with the stress of hard physical work, such evolutionary
change in man will take a long time. The only available
chance for bridging the existing gap in adequate
adaptability is the regular training of the organic power
through the familiar stress of physical exercise.*

— KASCH and BOYER
Adult Fitness

Your program must continue on a regular basis if you expect progress. Results, once achieved, are maintained by continuous exercise also. Your results will almost directly parallel your efforts.

Notes

1. Frank Vitale, *Individualized Exercise Programs* (Englewood Cliffs: Prentice-Hall, Inc., 1973), p. 76.
2. *Ibid.*, p. 79.
3. Harold B. Falls, Earl L. Wallis, and Gene A. Logan, *Foundations of Conditioning* (New York: Academic Press, 1970), p. 43.
4. *Ibid.*
5. Herbert A. deVries, *Physiology of Exercise* (Dubuque: Wm. C. Brown Company Publishers, 1974), p. 447.
6. Janet A. Wessel, *Movement Fundamentals* (Englewood Cliffs: Prentice-Hall, Inc., 1970), p. 74.
7. *Ibid.*
8. Vitale, *Individualized Exercise Programs*, pp. 78–79.
9. Phillip J. Rasch and Roger K. Burke. *Kinesiology and Applied Anatomy* (Philadelphia: Lea and Febiger, 1975), p. 436.
10. Leonard A. Larson and Herbert Michelman, *International Guide to Fitness and Health* (New York: Crow Publishers, Inc., 1973), p. 20.
11. Fred W. Kasch and John L. Boyer, *Adult Fitness* (Palo Alto: Mayfield Publishing Company, 1968), p. 13.
12. Larson and Michelman, *International Guide to Fitness and Health*, p. 25.

6 | ENDURANCE EXERCISE

"Aerobics" became a household word in the late 1960s, and the writings of Dr. Kenneth Cooper have made many of us realize that we have less than the ideal fitness level. Consider the term *physical fitness*. What does it mean to you?

The experts discuss physical fitness in reference to the heart and circulatory systems, using the terms *cardiovascular* and *cardiorespiratory* fitness, respectively. Cardiovascular and respiratory fitness means that the heart, circulatory system, and lungs are in good condition. These three can be thought of as the transportation system of the body. The heart with its pumping action propels the nutrient-carrying blood (nourished in part by oxygen from the lungs) through our circulatory system of arteries and veins. A weak transportation system will affect the entire body; a strong, properly conditioned system can be an excellent life insurance policy.

THE RESULTS OF INACTIVITY

When the transportation system is damaged or functioning improperly, a degree of cardiovascular disease has occurred. The latest statistics on heart disease have apparently led more and more persons to take up jogging, swimming, and bicycling in pursuit of improved health. Heart disease can be detected by an impairment of the blood supply to vital organs and other parts of the body. Inefficient blood supply to the heart, for instance, can lead

47

> *Physical activities that develop endurance are the "heart" of
> the exercise program. They are designed to improve both the
> capacity and efficiency of the cardiovascular and respiratory
> systems. Also, they are the types of exercises that are most
> useful in helping to control or reduce body weight.*
>
> — JACK WILMORE
> *Athletic Training and Physical Fitness*

to what is commonly called a heart attack; and poor blood circulation to the
brain can result in a stroke. Although these are not the only results of circulatory impairment, they are certainly among the most important ones to
those of us who want a long and active life.

THE BENEFITS OF ENDURANCE EXERCISE

The type of exercise that strengthens our transportation system has been
labeled cardiovascular endurance exercise, or simply endurance exercise.
As we can easily see, it is one of the most important parts of physical fitness.
Endurance is the ability to do continuous physical work, whether for pleasure or necessity; it could be called our "work capacity." Study the following possible benefits of endurance exercise, then weigh the relatively small
time investment against the advantages to be gained:

1. Exercise can increase the efficiency of the lungs and respiratory system
   thereby allowing the lungs to process more air with less effort and increase the amount of oxygen the body is able to utilize.
2. Exercise can increase the supply of blood to the heart by increasing the
   number of capillaries throughout the body and the size of the arteries in
   the heart as well as in the body. The result is a more efficient exchange of
   nutrients, oxygen, and waste products. Increased oxygen results in increased energy available during times of stress.
3. Exercise can enhance the development of collateral circulation, which
   means providing additional sources of blood supply to the heart.
   This would provide alternative pathways should blood vessels become
   clogged.
4. Exercise can result in increased efficiency of the heart, since training
   usually results in an increase in the size of the heart muscle and therefore
   an improvement in its pumping action. As we know, the effectiveness of
   pumps are generally closely related to their size. This means the heart
   will be able to pump a greater volume of blood with each beat.

5. Exercise can reduce the resting heart rate, which means more rest for the heart.[1]
6. Exercise may increase the body's fat tolerance which refers to the clearing of lipids from the bloodstream. When a high-fat meal is ingested, fat passes through the bloodstream where it is deposited in the liver, stored as adipose tissue (fat), or used. If we can clear fat quickly from the blood, we have a high fat tolerance.
7. Exercise can aid in reducing an obese or overweight condition by causing us to use more calories during our waking hours.

With these seven advantages of exercise in mind, it is easy to recognize the dependence of the various organs and systems of the body, one upon another. "Our most urgent need is for a continual supply of oxygen."[2] Strong lungs provide an increased supply of oxygen to the blood, a more efficient heart delivers more oxygen to the muscles, and stronger muscles can result in more vigorous activity, which in turn provides conditioning for both the lungs and the heart.[3]

THE GOAL OF ENDURANCE EXERCISE

We must subject our body to increased demands so that our tolerance of hard work and stress can be increased in order to improve our physical fitness level. We must force our heart to take on a progressively more difficult workload in order to increase its strength. The overload principle, as explained in Chapter 4, applies here.

The idea behind endurance exercise is to decrease the resting heart rate. This is accomplished by using the overload principle and increasing the workload of the heart through a controlled activity, such as the jogging program described later in this chapter. Controlled training through the use of the overload principle will cause your resting heart rate to decrease; this can be seen from the low heart rates of cross-country runners. As the resting heart rate decreases, the heart begins to pump blood more efficiently, and our work capacity increases. It seems to be a general rule of nature that the slower the heart rate, the longer the life-span. Consider that an elephant, who may live for one hundred years, has a heart rate of 25 beats per minute, whereas the mouse, who may live for only one year, has a rate of 600 to 700 beats per minute. For optimum health, it is desirable to develop the slowest resting heart rate possible.

COUNTING THE PULSE

Pulse rate is the most practical measure for determining our workload during activity, as well as for testing the effectiveness of our endurance program. It will also indicate whether or not our exercise program or workload has been too intense or strenuous. By counting your pulse during activity, you may determine the extent of your workload and adjust or stop your activity accordingly. Recording your resting pulse rate over a period of time will indicate the success of your exercise program, and keeping a record of your pulse after activity will tell you if your program is too demanding. Your pulse rate should return to its average resting rate within 30 minutes after the workout; if it does not, you are exercising too hard.

The first thing to remember in taking your pulse is to use your fingers for feeling the pulse, instead of your thumb. This is because the thumb carries its own pulse, which makes it difficult to count accurately. The pulse may be taken more effectively at one of three areas of the body: (1) on the wrist just below the base of the thumb; (2) inside the bend of the elbow; and (3) on either of the large carotid arteries, which run on each frontal side of the neck.

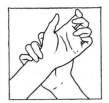 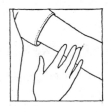 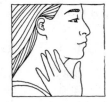

The resting pulse rate should be taken after at least 30 minutes of restful activity, such as sitting, reading, watching television, or relaxing. You should take it and write it down on a regular basis in order to establish a good record.

The active pulse rate should be taken immediately after stopping the exercise activity. You should count for only 10 seconds and then multiply the number of beats by six (to equal a minute), because the pulse rate decreases very quickly after activity. To insure that the pulse rate is within acceptable limits, the pulse should be taken several times during the activity phase of your exercise program. When this is called for, stop during the endurance activity, estimate your pulse using the 10-second count, then resume the activity.

A recovery pulse rate should be taken within 10 to 30 minutes after ending your workout. If this pulse has not returned to your resting rate by the end of 30 minutes, make your next workout less strenuous, and check the results in the same way.

It is important to assume the same position when taking each pulse count, because the pulse rate is different in standing, sitting, and lying positions. The active pulse count—taken while exercising or immediately thereafter—should be taken in a standing position, but the recovery and resting counts are best taken in a lying or sitting position.

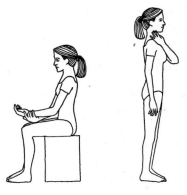

Before you start your endurance program, you should prepare yourself as follows:

1. See which of the areas of the body (wrist, elbow, neck) give you the strongest pulse.
2. Take your pulse in each of the positions: lying down, sitting, and standing. Use a 15-second pulse count and multiply by 4 to determine the pulse rate for a minute.
3. Use the Heart Rate Count Chart, found in Appendix B, to determine your appropriate present heart-rate status.

PLANNING YOUR PROGRAM

As you begin to plan your endurance program, it is important to realize that all activities are not equal in value. Only those exercises requiring continuous, vigorous movement will contribute to cardiovascular fitness. Specifically, in order to obtain significant improvement (training effect) in the cardiovascular system, the following three criteria must be met:

1. Intensity: the exercise must be vigorous enough to produce a specific sustained pulse rate.[4] (See Appendix C.)
2. Duration: the exercise must be continued at this level for 20 to 30 minutes.[5]
3. Frequency: the exercise must be performed regularly (every other day).[6]

The progressive jogging program described below gradually incorporates these three criteria.

STAGE ONE This is your beginning program, which requires jogging three days a week for three weeks, with each session lasting approximately 15 minutes. You should never go more than two days between sessions.

GOAL: To work toward jogging continuously for 3 minutes.

ACTIVITY:
1. Begin with a warm-up walk for 2 to 3 minutes.
2. Alternate jogging and walking for 10 minutes. Remember, you must continue this part for 10 minutes, so don't wear yourself out in the first 2 minutes by going too fast.
3. End with a 2 or 3 minute cool-down walk.

SUGGESTIONS:
1. The walk in the warm-up should begin slowly and build up to a brisk pace toward the end of the 3 minutes. Do just the opposite in the cool-down.
2. The jog-walk-jog phase (activity 2) can be repeated as many times as necessary to equal 10 minutes. Use a brisk walk in this phase.
3. As you progress, shorten the walking time and lengthen the jogging time.

STAGE TWO This is where you will begin to apply the intensity, duration, and frequency criteria listed above. You should stay at this stage for two weeks, working out every other day for approximately 20 minutes.

GOAL A pulse rate within the training range (150 beats per minute, but not more than 180).

ACTIVITY
1. Warm up for 2 minutes with a slow to brisk walk.
2. Alternate jogging and walking for 15 minutes.
3. End with a cool-down, a brisk and then a slow walk.

SUGGESTIONS
1. Use a 10-second pulse count and work towards achieving a minimum pulse count for 10 seconds.
2. Try to keep the pulse between the maximum and minimum for 10 seconds.
3. Stop periodically, about every 2 to 3 minutes, to count your pulse.

STAGE THREE	During this stage, the maintenance stage, you will add the third criteria—frequency—to your program. This will mean working out every other day for 20 to 30 minutes.
GOAL	To keep the activity pulse rate within the training zone (between 25 and 30 seconds) for a 10-second count and to work out regularly.
ACTIVITY	1. Begin each workout with a 2- to 3-minute warm-up walk.
	2. Continue the alternated jogging and walking for 15 minutes, and work slowly up to 20 minutes.
	3. End with cool-down walk of 2 to 3 minutes.
SUGGESTIONS	1. Work gradually toward jogging for the entire 20 minutes.
	2. Continue counting your pulse periodically as you jog, in order to keep it between 25 to 30 beats for 10 seconds.
	3. Add 2 to 5 minutes of flexibility exercises after your cool-down. Use the exercises described in Chapter 7 and do them as instructed. They will stretch the muscles that have become tight and tense from running.
	4. As you progress, you will find that it will take more effort to maintain the minimum activity pulse rate. You must then increase your running speed accordingly.

This is only one of many possible cardiovascular conditioning programs, and although jogging is probably the most convenient method, it is by no means the only successful one. Perhaps you might enjoy bicycling, swimming, jumping rope, or some another vigorous activity. These activities can be effective alternatives to running—provided that you use the three endurance criteria and apply the overload principle. You can use the minimum activity pulse rate count for any of these other activities. You might also want to try Dr. Cooper's carefully devised program, which covers many endurance activities.[7]

WARMING UP AND COOLING DOWN

As discussed in Chapter 4, each type of exercise should begin with a warm-up and end with a cooling-down period. The same is true of endurance exercise. You must allow time for the body to shift from resting to vigorous movement, and vice-versa. As we have said, this will help prevent muscle soreness, injuries, and the possible pooling of blood in the extremities. Cold drinks, hot showers, steamy rooms, and particularly saunas should be avoided until you have stopped perspiring (which usually means from 5 to 15 minutes).[8]

ONCE IS NOT ENOUGH

Ideally, endurance programs should be performed daily, but good results can be obtained from sessions three times a week if they are distributed evenly throughout the week, with a maximum of two days between sessions. After 48 hours, a significant reduction in fitness occurs. Research has shown that a person who is sedentary for only three days will lose approximately 5 percent of his or her original conditioning.[9] A month of inactivity can result in an 80 percent conditioning loss.[10]

HELPFUL HINTS

1. Too much exertion will cause excessive fatigue, which is likely to create a negative attitude toward endurance exercise. So take it easy in the beginning, and add a little more with each exercise session.
2. Strenuous exercise within an hour before or after eating a meal can interfere with digestion, because the blood supply is diverted from the digestive system to the muscles being used. Light exercise does not alter the digestive process, except to cause the stomach to empty a bit more quickly.
3. The intensity and duration of your workouts should be shortened during extreme weather conditions—below 40 degrees F or above 85 degrees F—unless you have access to a space with a controlled temperature, such as a gymnasium.
4. During the walking phase of your exercise, your walk should be brisk rather than slow. Use slow walking only at the beginning of the warm-up phase and the end of the cool-down phase.
5. Jogging is a slow form of running and should be continued at a moderate, even pace.
6. You should jog or run only on grass or soft ground. Running on concrete sidewalks, hard pavement, or even asphalt can cause injury to the body. It is also suggested that you confine running to level areas. Running on hills takes special training and skill.
7. The clothing worn during exercise should be loose-fitting and comfortable. An inexpensive cotton "sweatsuit" is desirable on cool days;

otherwise shorts or pants and a loose shirt are acceptable. During cool weather the legs should be covered. Don't try to save money when purchasing running shoes. Buy them at a good sporting goods store and expect to pay up to twenty dollars or more for a good pair.

8. Cigarettes and coffee can alter your pulse rate during exercise. If you smoke or drink coffee, or both, it might be a good idea to cut down on your use of them considerably, and to eliminate them entirely one to two hours before you start your endurance exercise.

9. Alcohol and drugs, even antibiotics, should not be mixed with an endurance program. Recorded deaths have been caused when running under the influence of antibiotics. If you are taking antibiotics or other medicines, consult your doctor about your activity.

10. A physical examination should be a prerequisite to any exercise program.

TURNING BACK THE CLOCK

Although chronological aging is inevitable, physical age may vary as much as thirty years. Almost all biological processes begin to slow down after the age of thirty. However, Dr. Herbert de Vries, in his research on Leisure World residents, concludes: "Exercise can bring about a renewal of the heart function on older subjects. Conservatively speaking, we saw a reduction of ten to twenty years in their heart's oxygen transport capacity even if they had been relatively inactive for years."[11]

It's never too late to begin walking or running that road back to health. But wouldn't it be wonderful if all of our children were taught at an early age to enjoy the benefits of good health and physical fitness? First, and most important for all of us, is to set a good example, so that all those who come in contact with us will be affected by our effort. That is the best way to spread the word and help make your world a better and healthier place in which to live.

Notes

1. Robert V. Hockey, *Physical Fitness, the Pathway to Healthful Living* (St. Louis: The C. V. Mosby Company, 1977), p. 142.

2. W. W. Tuttle and Byron A. Schottelius, *Textbook of Physiology* (St. Louis: The C. V. Mosby Company, 1969), p. 303.

3. Frank Vitale, *Individualized Fitness* (Englewood Cliffs: Prentice-Hall, Inc., 1973), p. 40.

4. Leonore R. Zohman, *Beyond Diet: Exercise Your Way to Fitness and Heart Health* (CPC International, Inc., 1974), p. 15.

5. *Ibid.*, p. 18.

6. *Ibid.*, pp. 15–19.

7. Kenneth H. Cooper, *The New Aerobics* (New York: Bantam Books, 1978), pp. 52–114.

8. *Ibid.,* p. 38.

9. Laurence Moorehouse, *Total Fitness* (St. Louis: Simon and Schuster, 1975), p. 37.

10. *Ibid.,* p. 59.

11. Herbert A. deVries, *Vigor Regained* (Englewood Cliffs: Prentice-Hall, Inc., 1974), p. 37.

7 | *FLEXIBILITY EXERCISE*

Decreased flexibility may, more than any other factor, limit the amount of enthusiasm or motivation that a person has for exercise.

KENNETH LERSTEN
Physiology and Physical Conditioning

Most great athletes have great flexibility, which accounts for their graceful, well-coordinated movements. This flexibility, which is a result of exercise, is not only important to athletes but also valuable to all persons, especially as they age.

FACTORS AFFECTING FLEXIBILITY

Inactivity usually results in inflexibility, which is why active people tend to be more flexible than inactive people. Therefore it is important for us to take appropriate exercises in order to keep our bodies limber. Since this type of exercise is not common to the activities of everyday living, we must plan to engage regularly in flexibility exercises.

As we age, the quality of elasticity tends to disappear from ligaments, tendons, and muscles.[1] Compare the free, unrestricted movement of a child with that of an older person. You will see a vast difference in their movement capabilities.

Other factors affecting flexibility are sex, body build or figure, obesity, and occupational or recreational habits. To give one example, women tend to be more flexible than men. But it has yet to be proved whether this is a physical sex difference or the result of previous environmental adaptation. Wearing high-heeled shoes and boots, for instance, can result in inflexibility in the back and in the legs. Participation in certain sports, habitual movement patterns, and job activities can cause specific patterns of flexibility or inflexibility.[2]

> *Though the characteristics which distinguish physical activity from other types of activity would seem to be self-evident, one soon realizes that human movement is, indeed, a highly complex phenomenon.*
>
> —R. B. ALDERMAN
> *Psychological Behavior in Sport*

Lifestyle, then, is very important in determining the length of our active years. We must become aware of the types of bodily movement caused by our lifestyle and make an effort to correct the deficiencies where flexibility is concerned.

THE IMPORTANCE OF REMAINING FLEXIBLE

The ability to move freely and easily and without pain is clearly important to all of us. Flexibility also helps to prevent injury to joints, which is especially important to athletes and to all of us as we grow older.

A flexible muscle can stretch further before tearing or injury occurs. Flexible people are less susceptible to sprains, strains, and dislocations.

Improved posture and relief of menstrual cramps and lower back pain are some of the most common benefits of increasing one's flexibility.[3] There are also many psychological benefits. If we are able to move freely, we usually look better and as a result feel better. We gain grace and coordination, as well as faster reaction time, the enjoyment of which is not reserved only for the athlete. Whether we are male or female, athlete or spectator, improved flexibility can give us a new attitude toward living.

PHYSIOLOGICAL STRUCTURE

An understanding of the relationship among muscles, bones, and joints is necessary to fully comprehend the benefits of flexibility exercise. The different bones of our body are connected at various points, which are called joints.

A *joint* is the junction of two or more bones, held together by ligaments, lubricated by bursae (cushions between bones), and bound by tendons.[4] Joints, also called *articulations,* are either movable or immovable. Our primary concern is with the movable joints, because flexibility depends upon the use of movable joints. The bones that meet to form movable joints are covered by cartilage and held together by ligaments.[5] The bursae, which are composed of a synovial membrane outside and fluid inside, lubricate the joints.

Muscles are connected to bone and cartilage in the joint area by tendons and are covered by a membrane called *fascia.*

Tendons are fibrous cords of considerable strength and have no elasticity.[6]

It's not short arms that prevent you from touching your toes, but a lack of flexibility in the muscles of the legs.

—CHARLES T. KUNTZELMAN
Physical Fitness Encyclopedia

Flexibility, or range of movement, is determined by all of these— ligaments, tendons, muscles, and muscle sheaths (fascia). Because ligaments are naturally pliant and flexible and tendons lack elasticity, it appears that flexibility exercises have the greatest effect on muscles and fascia.

JOINT AND MUSCLE ACTION

Joints are capable of rotating, swinging, and gliding movements. When a joint moves, muscles must both stretch and contract. This action is called flexion and extension. Individuals differ in the degree of joint articulation or flexibility they have, because they differ in muscular as well as in ligament or tendon structure; some persons have shorter muscles, ligaments, and tendons. Also, the degree of joint movement will vary within the various joints in your own body. Usually the one arm used the most will be the less flexible one, because more time has been spent flexing it than extending it. This indicates the importance of both strength and flexibility in a muscle.

THE STRETCH REFLEX

The stretch (myotatic) reflex can actually inhibit the process of becoming limber. When one set of muscles extend, the opposite set of muscles will contract. This is natural and involuntary; it will happen even when you concentrate on preventing it. Therefore, in order to improve flexibility, *we must cause the contracting set of muscles to relax while we extend the opposite set of muscles.* If relaxation in the muscles opposite the action does not occur, movement will not result.[7] The myotatic stretch reflex appears to be a protective mechanism that tends to occur most frequently in rapid, uncontrolled stretching actions.[8] Since the opposing muscle group is actively engaged in resisting an active stretch, yet weakens and "lets go," a muscle strain or other injury is likely to occur.

BALLISTIC VERSUS STATIC STRETCH   Ballistic movements are rapid, jerking actions, which allow for little control. Static stretching, on the other hand, is slow and steady. Research has shown that a static (nonmoving) pull allows for greater relaxation of the opposing muscle group and results in greater improvement in flexibility with less chance for injury to a muscle.[9]

Ballistic or bouncing movements produce an intense stretch reflex that can allow for over-stretching—if the ballistic movements are stronger than the protective stretch reflex. In addition, ballistic stretching can cause severe soreness, whereas static stretching can prevent much of the soreness associated with flexibility exercises. As a matter of fact, static stretching can be an aid in the relief of muscle soreness caused by overexercise.[10]

> *Concentration is the supreme art because no art can be achieved without it. By learning to concentrate, one develops a skill that can heighten performance in every aspect of his life. The concentrated mind does not admit distractions, externally or internally; it is totally engrossed in the object of concentration.*
>
> *—W. TIMOTHY CALLWEY*
> *The Inner Game of Tennis*

USING THE STATIC STRETCH   Concentration is of utmost importance when employing static stretching. You must coordinate your mind with your body and learn to feel the movement in your muscles. In a sense, you must *think* with your muscles as well as your mind in order to develop an awareness of your body; of how it moves and how it feels when it moves. The following preparation exercises will help you begin this process:

1. Bend forward at the waist while standing with legs together. Be certain not to lock or hyperextend your knees. Let your upper body and arms hang

loosely toward the floor. In this position, concentrate on how your muscles feel as gravity stretches the muscles in your legs and lower back. Lean forward over the balls of your feet, almost to the point of losing balance and falling over forward. Stop at that point and stay in that position. Try to stay in this position for 30 seconds. During this time, try to describe to yourself the

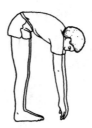

sensations you are feeling within your muscles and body. Where are your hands in relation to the floor? Do you feel pain, discomfort, or another feeling? Are your hands moving closer to the floor? This is an excellent exercise to add to any warm-up program and is especially good as a warm-up for your flexibility program.

2. Sit facing a wall with your legs out straight in front of you and the bottoms of your feet flat against the wall. Lean forward and try to touch the wall with your fingertips while your legs are straight. See if you can touch the

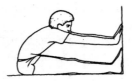

wall without bending your knees. If you can, place as much of your hands against the wall as you can and see if you can walk your hands down the wall until your palms are flat against the wall directly above your toes with the heel of your hand touching your toes. Hold the position where you must stop for 30 seconds if you can. If you are not able to reach the wall with your fingertips, estimate the number of inches they are from the wall. Concentrate on holding them as close to the wall as possible, without moving, for 30 seconds. This is another exercise to add to a warm-up program.

These are exercises in concentration as well as in flexibility. Practice them until you can achieve a floor touch in Exercise 1 and a wall touch in Exercise 2.

When doing flexibility exercises, all movements to and from the stretch position should be slow, deliberate, and controlled. Pull slowly into position, hold the position for the required number of seconds, then release. You should pull past the point of mild discomfort each time. If the pull is too vigorous, the muscles will tense, which will work against the achievement of flexibility by activating the stretch reflex discussed previously. Pulling too lightly will not place an overload on the muscle group being exercised, so the increase in flexibility will be minimal.

FACTS RELATED TO FLEXIBILITY

Before planning your flexibility program, it is important to be aware of the following factors regarding flexibility and to keep them in mind as you plan and continue to work on flexibility:

1. Flexibility is more likely to be improved when there is an elevation in the internal temperature of the body.[11]

2. In order for increases in range of motion to occur, the stretch must be carried to the point of moderate pain and slightly beyond.[12]

3. Flexibility is gained by the application of increased effort at regular intervals.[13]

4. Flexibility exercises should be done slowly and under control without developing momentum.[14]

5. More intensity is required to increase the range of motion than to maintain it.[15]

6. The maintenance of adequate flexibility appears to depend upon the amount and intensity of movement of the body parts through complete ranges of motion every day.[16]

7. The areas of the body requiring the most emphasis in terms of flexibility are the thigh, hip region, trunk or back, and the chest.

PLANNING YOUR PROGRAM

The flexibility program which follows is a progressive plan incorporating the factors just listed. Recommended exercises follow the program.

Warm-Up   A warm-up is critical to your flexibility program. Since improvement in flexibility is closely related to an increase in internal body temperature, most authorities suggest that a flexibility program should immediately follow an endurance program.[17] If this is impossible, spend at least 5 to 10 minutes of running in place, jumping rope, or stair-climbing prior to each flexibility session.

Your warm-up has served its purpose when you begin to perspire lightly.

STAGE ONE

Stay at this introductory level for three weeks. The initial stage of a daily flexibility exercise routine will last approximately 5 minutes, excluding your warm-up.

GOAL

To become adjusted to a daily routine and to incorporate the static stretch method of exercise.

ACTIVITY

1. Use Exercises one through six.
2. Hold each stretch for 15 seconds.
3. Rest for 30 seconds between each exercise.
4. Do each exercise only one time.

SUGGESTIONS

1. Pull past the point of first pain and hold each position at that point.
2. If it is too difficult to use a watch or clock for counting, count "one, one thousand; two, one thousand; three, one thousand," and so on.
3. Release each exercise position slowly.
4. Don't forget to warm up.

STAGE TWO

The application of increased effort is applied in this stage. Remain at this level for three weeks while continuing to work out every day.

GOAL

To concentrate on increasing and holding the stretch position and the amount of effort expended.

ACTIVITY

1. Use Exercises one through ten.
2. Hold each stretch for 30 seconds.
3. Rest for 30 seconds between each exercise.
4. Do each exercise only one time.

SUGGESTIONS

1. Concentrate on the stretch and the body position.
2. Take care to assume the correct position.
3. Pull slowly and release slowly.
4. Remember the importance of warm-up.

STAGE THREE

The rest period in this stage will be decreased, while the hold will be increased in the stretch position. Stay at this level for four weeks. For added benefit and more rapid results, work out twice a day.

GOAL	To maintain a one-minute, static stretch hold in each exercise position, which results in an increase in intensity.
ACTIVITY	1. Use Exercises one through ten. 2. Hold each stretch for 30 seconds. 3. Rest for 15 seconds between each exercise. 4. Do each exercise only once.
SUGGESTIONS	1. Now that you are used to the exercises, you might want to try a watch or clock for counting. 2. Music will help ease the discomfort. 3. Pull as far as you can on each exercise. 4. Warm-up comes first.
STAGE FOUR	Results should be adequate by now. If you wish to achieve increased flexibility from this point, stay on Stage Three until you are satisfied with the results, then change to this stage. Stage Four should be continued as long as you wish to maintain an adequate level of flexibility.
GOAL	To establish a maintenance program for flexibility.
ACTIVITY	1. Work out daily or twice a day. 2. Use all ten exercises. 3. Hold each stretch position for 15 seconds.
SUGGESTIONS	1. Stretch as far as you can with each exercise position. 2. Ease in and out of each stretch. 3. If your exercise program must be interrupted for some length of time, two weeks or longer, return to a previous stage and work up to this point again. You will not have to return to Stage One unless you are out of exercise for six weeks or longer. Flexibility is not lost as readily as strength or endurance. Use your own judgment and return to the level that seems adequate.

HELPFUL HINTS

1. Don't forget to warm up as directed before each flexibility exercise session.
2. Wear loose, comfortable clothing.

3. Go without shoes if you can.

4. Wear a sweatsuit if you can afford to purchase one. Department stores sell the cotton type at reasonable prices.

5. Use a mat, rug, or carpeted floor for exercising rather than a hard floor.

6. There is no "right" time for exercise. Two "wrong" times, however, are directly before retiring at night, and right after eating.

7. Make flexibility exercise a part of each and every day. Don't miss an exercise session unless you have to.

8. If time is a problem, combine endurance and flexibility workouts. You will be adding only a few minutes to your endurance workout.

9. Lateral trunk flexion or trunk rotation should always precede forward flexion of the trunk.[18] This helps release tension in the muscles. For this reason, always do Exercise One first.

THE EXERCISES

Exercise One

OBJECTIVE — This exercise is for the side of the abdominal area and the outside of the thigh (upper leg).

DIRECTIONS — Stand with your feet shoulder-width apart with one arm up and one arm down at side. Bend to the side, toward the arm hanging down, until you feel discomfort in the stretch. Hold for the required number of seconds, then exchange arm positions and repeat on the opposite side.

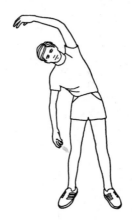

Exercise Two

OBJECTIVE This is a waist exercise designed to stretch the trunk area.

DIRECTIONS Stand with feet shoulder-width apart and upper arms extended at shoulder level. Elbows should be bent so that fists can touch at chest level. Turn as far as you can to the right and hold. Repeat the rotation to the left and hold.

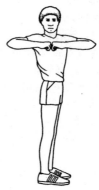

Exercise Three

OBJECTIVE This is an exercise for the area around the shoulder and the upper arm.

DIRECTIONS Stand with feet shoulder-width apart and one arm reaching around behind the body and upward toward the shoulders. Try to touch fingertips or clasp hands. Reach as far as you can and hold. Change arm position and repeat.

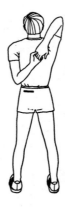

Exercise Four

OBJECTIVE

This exercise is designed to improve flexibility in the lower back and legs.

DIRECTIONS

Stand with feet slightly apart while bending forward at the waist by bending your knees until you can place the palms of your hands flat on the floor. You should be almost in a squat position. Keep the palms on the floor as you straighten your legs until the stretch becomes uncomfortable in the legs and lower back. Hold this position. Do not overextend (hyperextend) your knees. They should always be very slightly bent. As your improved flexibility allows you to achieve maximum stretch in this position, change the hand position to holding on to the ankles and pull your head as close to your knees as you can and hold.

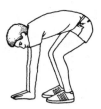

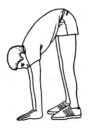 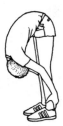

Exercise Five

OBJECTIVE   This is an exercise designed to stretch the gastrocnemius muscle in the calf of the lower leg.

DIRECTIONS   Stand approximately three to four feet from and facing a wall. Lean forward toward the wall with your arms outstretched in front of you while keeping your body straight until your palms are flat against the wall supporting your body weight. Keep your heels against the floor at all times throughout the exercise. Bend your elbows to increase body lean until the stretch in the calf almost lifts your heels from the floor. Hold this position.

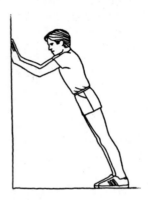

Exercise Six

OBJECTIVE   This exercise stretches the muscles in the front and back of the thigh.

DIRECTIONS   Sit with one leg extended, toe pointed, and the opposite leg bent at the knee and behind you. Lean forward while keeping your head and chin up and try to pull your chest to your knee as you grasp as far down the leg as you can. Hold just past the first point of pain. Repeat on the opposite leg.

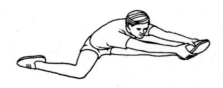

Exercise Seven

OBJECTIVE
This is an excellent stretching exercise for the groin area and the inner portion of the upper thigh.

DIRECTIONS
Sit with legs in front of your body, the knees bent, and the bottoms of your feet touching. Grasp your toes with both hands and pull your chest toward your heels until you feel discomfort in the stretch. Hold this position. Keep your head and chin up as you pull down.

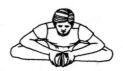

Exercise Eight

OBJECTIVE
This exercise is for the improvement of flexibility in the shoulder, chest, and upper arm areas.

DIRECTIONS
Stand with feet shoulder-width apart and arms behind you while clasping hands securely. Bend forward at the waist while keeping arms straight and pull them as far over your body as you can. Hold this position.

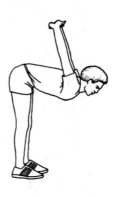

Exercise Nine

OBJECTIVE

This exercise is in three positions and is excellent for improving flexibility in the lower back, thigh, and groin.

DIRECTIONS

Sit, with back straight and legs in a wide-stride position in front of you. The toes should be pointed and the feet and legs rotated backward. Don't let the feet fall inward. Pull the chin toward the right toe as you pull the chest toward your right knee. Hold in this position. Repeat on the opposite leg. Then grasp each leg as close to the ankle as possible and pull forward. Hold the head and chin up and pull your chest toward the floor. Try to widen your stride a little each time you exercise.

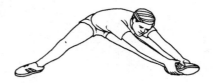

Exercise Ten

OBJECTIVE

This exercise is for the improvement of flexibility in the ankle and foot area.

DIRECTIONS

Stand with feet apart. Lift one foot and roll it over and forward so that you can press down on the top of the foot. Press until the stretch is severe and hold. Repeat on the other foot.

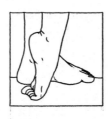

Notes

1. Herbert A. deVries, *Physiology of Exercise* (Dubuque: Wm. C. Brown Company Publishers, 1974), pp. 240–41.

2. Phillip J. Rasch and Roger K. Burke, *Kinesiology and Applied Anatomy* (Philadelphia: Lea and Febiger, 1975), pp. 37–38.

3. *Ibid.*

4. B. J. Brown, *Complete Guide to the Prevention and Treatment of Athletic Injuries* (West Nyack: Parker Publishing Company, 1972), p. 56.

5. Henry Gray, *Gray's Anatomy,* T. Pickering Pick and Robert Howden, eds. (Philadelphia: Running Press, 1901), p. 219–20.

6. *Ibid.*, p. 296.

7. Harold B. Falls, Earl A. Wallis, and Gene A. Logan, *Foundations of Conditioning* (New York: Academic Press, 1970), p. 51.

8. *Ibid.*

9. Carl E. Klafs and Daniel P. Arnheim, *Modern Principles of Athletic Training* (St. Louis: The C. V. Mosby Company, 1969), p. 53.

10. DeVries, *Physiology of Exercise,* pp. 436–37.

11. *Ibid.*, p. 440.

12. Falls, Wallis, and Logan, *Foundations of Conditioning,* p. 177.

13. Gene A. Logan, *Adaptations of Muscular Activity* (Belmont: Wadsworth Publishing Company, Inc., 1964), p. 176.

14. *Ibid.*, p. 177.

15. Falls, Wallis, and Logan, p. 54.

16. *Ibid.*, p. 55.

17. Logan, *Adaptations of Muscular Activity.*

18. Fred W. Kasch and John L. Boyer, *Adult Fitness: Principles and Practice* (Palo Alto: Mayfield Publishing Company, 1968), p. 41.

8 | *STRENGTH EXERCISE*

There are 656 skeletal muscles in the body. Each of these has a specialized function to perform. Together, they make up 42 percent of the total weight in the male and 36 percent in the female.

JAMES A. BALEY
Illustrated Guide to Developing Athletic Strength, Power, and Agility

Often we hear the human body compared to a machine. Like an engine, muscles give power and force to the body. Unlike most engines, however, our muscles do not wear out with use but instead become more efficient. Strength is the foundation upon which all other processes of our body depend. When muscles are weak, the quality of our physical and mental performance decreases. Although muscular strength is most often associated with athletes, all of us must possess a minimum of strength merely in order to stand upright. The more strength we possess, the greater is our potential for good posture. Improved posture enhances our appearance as well as our functioning.

ENDURANCE VERSUS STRENGTH

As explained in Chapter 6, one of the criteria for endurance is the ability to repeat movements over a long period of time at a less than maximum level. In contrast, strength is usually defined as the maximum amount of force a muscle can exert once and once only.[1] Accordingly, strength exercises emphasize few repetitions of maximum force, usually against a type of resis-

73

tance. When the repetitions exceed ten, the activity begins to take on the aspects of endurance as opposed to strength exercise.[2]

Because of the repetitive nature of endurance activity, more energy is necessary to sustain it than is required in strength development. However, the development of strength requires the cardiovascular system to supply the increased oxygen necessary for production of maximum power,[3] and the cardiovascular system is developed by endurance exercise.

> Man has shown a perpetual curiosity about the organs of locomotion in his own body and in those of other creatures. Indeed, some of the earliest scientific experiments known to us concerned muscle and its functions.
>
> —J. V. BASMAJIAN
> *Muscles Alive*

MUSCULAR GROWTH

A muscle is a group of contractile fibers covered by connective tissue. When a muscle is stimulated, each fiber contracts individually at maximum power or it does not contract at all. The number of fibers within a muscle is dictated by its size and action. Exercise causes the muscle to grow in size but not in the number of its fibers. Exercise also causes an increase in the number of capillaries within the muscle, as a result of the need to deliver extra fuel to the muscle.[4]

STRENGTH IMPROVEMENT

The most rapid increases in strength occur between the ages of twelve and nineteen and begin to level off at around thirty years of age. We are at our strongest between ages twenty and thirty. Fortunately, however, the decrease in strength after maturity is very gradual, and even by the age of sixty the loss usually does not exceed 10 to 20 percent of the maximum. The decline in strength can be attributed to a decrease in the quantity of muscle tissue rather than to qualitative changes.[5] Thus it seems reasonable to conclude that the continuance of strength exercises as we get older will decrease the inevitable loss of strength during aging.[6]

STRENGTH DEVELOPMENT

We perform strength-developing activities every day. An example would be lifting bags of groceries or climbing stairs. Because our environment itself provides fewer and fewer strength-developing activities, however, it is important to have a well-planned set of exercises that we perform at regular intervals to ensure proper strength development and maintenance.

The four methods of strength development are isometrics, isotonics, isokinetics, and weight training.

Isometrics caught the public eye back in the 1920s with Charles Atlas and his program of "dynamic tension." His was an isometric system involving muscular contractions with very little movement in the joints. Isometric exercise consists of contracting a muscle or muscle group against an immovable resistance, with relatively no movement occurring in the joint area as a result.[7] (A simple example would be pushing the palms of the hands hard against each other.) The process could be described as an irresistible force meeting an immovable object.

Isotonic movements contain two types of muscular contractions, concentric and eccentric. In concentric contraction, the muscle visibly shortens and develops tension to move a given resistance; in eccentric contraction, the muscle develops tension and lengthens.[8] In other words, an isotonic movement occurs when muscles contract and shorten, resulting in actual movement of the involved parts of the body.

Isokinetic exercise is a method of exercising in which the resistance to the muscle remains constant throughout the full range of movement.[9] This is accomplished through the use of a device or machine which, when pulled or pushed, adjusts to the force of the movement.

Weight training is probably the most widely used method of strength development today. This term describes a process of lifting weights, such as dumbbells, barbells, or the use of multiple-weight machines.

Weightlifting is a term used to describe a competitive weightlifting sport. The term weight training is used to describe a conditioning program whose objectives and end results will be applied in a match or athletic performance.

— ANTHONY A. ANNARINO
Developmental Conditioning for Physical Education and Athletics

---

WHICH PROGRAM TO USE

Each method of strength development has its advantages and disadvantages. For example, isometric exercises do not require much time or the use of any equipment, but there is no improvement in the range of movement of the joint, so we can probably assume that flexibility will not be improved—and could possibly be decreased. Isometric exercises are quite simple and cause very little fatigue; however, there can be a sudden rise in blood pressure during a maximum contraction, which might not cause problems for the young but could be potentially dangerous for older, less fit adults.[10]

Isotonic exercises, often called calisthenics, do not always result in maximum strength gains. Although it is true that exercises such as sit-ups and push-ups overload the participating muscles, thereby improving strength, every individual is operating at a different overload, so that it is difficult to anticipate the rate of improvement.[11] Because they do not require the use of equipment and are excellent for use with groups, calisthenics are probably the most widely used form of exercise.

> The first known weight-trained individual in history was Milo of Crotona, a Greek wrestler in the ancient days. . . . The training approach he chose was to daily lift a young calf across his shoulders and walk around a large stadium bearing the extra weight. Naturally, as the bullock grew older and heavier, Milo grew more powerful until he was acknowledged as the strongest man in the ancient world. . . . Milo's strength-building system was a crude form of progressive resistance exercise, or what we now call weight training.
>
> —BILL REYNOLDS
> *Complete Weight Training*

Weight training is the most efficient and effective form of strength-developing exercise. Its drawbacks are that it requires the use of additional equipment which can be cumbersome to the traveler or apartment dweller, and which, of course, costs money. Even if you do not buy the equipment yourself, the fees for using an established gym might be prohibitive.

Nevertheless, weight training remains the best single way to pursue strength development.

Isokinetic exercises, though an effective form of exercise, also involve the use of equipment and machines, which in some cases have not been satisfactory when used by large groups. Isokinetic exercises can be a valuable supplement to an exercise program, but good equipment is quite expensive.[12]

In view of the above, the best strength-development program is a combination of the different types of exercise, incorporating those which best meet your needs at any particular time. Use isometric exercises when you are traveling, and calisthenic exercises for preliminary strength building, as a warm-up to a weight-training program, and in combination with a weight-training program. If you are fortunate enough to be able to afford the equipment or have access to a gym, you will be able to use all types of strength-building exercises. Isometric, isotonic, and weight-training programs are presented below. Isokinetic exercises can be obtained where equipment is available.

AN ISOMETRIC EXERCISE PROGRAM

The isometric exercise program has only one stage. The exercises presented below are to be performed once only, with maximum effort. For added benefit, repeat the entire sequence of exercises.

ACTIVITY
1. Hold each position for 10 seconds while exerting maximum effort.
2. Rest for no longer than 15 seconds between exercises.
3. Perform each exercise one time.
4. Perform the exercises in the order listed.

SUGGESTIONS
1. Breathe normally during muscular contractions.
2. Maximum effort means to contract your muscles just as hard as you can.
3. The program can be repeated as many times during a day as you desire.

Exercise One

OBJECTIVE

This is an exercise to strengthen the arms and shoulders.

DIRECTIONS

Stand with your back about ten inches from a solid wall. Your feet should be shoulder-width apart and your arms should be held down at the sides of your body with palms flat against the wall. Using the wall for resistance, push hard against it while trying to pull your shoulder blades together. Hold this position for 10 seconds.

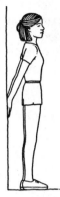

Exercise Two

OBJECTIVE

This exercise is to strengthen the muscles of the back, the abdominals, and the muscles of the seat (gluteal region).

DIRECTIONS

Stand with your back against, and your feet only a few inches from, a solid wall. Your knees should be slightly bent with arms down at your sides. While contracting your abdominal muscles (tummy area), press your shoulders, small of back, and seat as hard against the wall as you can. Hold this position for 10 seconds.

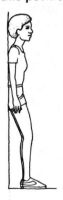

Exercise Three

OBJECTIVE

This is an exercise for strengthening the legs.

DIRECTIONS

Sit in an upright chair and cross your left ankle over and in front of your right ankle. Your knees should be bent with both feet flat on the floor. Stabilize your left ankle as you press your right ankle hard against it. Hold for 10 seconds. Recross ankles with right ankle in front and repeat a 10-second hold.

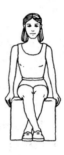

Exercise Four

OBJECTIVE

This is an exercise to strengthen the muscles of the neck region.

DIRECTIONS

Lie on your back on the floor with knees bent and arms at sides, palms against floor. Try to press your neck hard against the floor. Hold this position for 10 seconds.

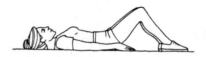

Exercise Five

OBJECTIVE
This exercise is designed to strengthen the muscles of the abdominal region.

DIRECTIONS
Lie on your back on the floor with legs extended and arms at your sides with palms against the floor. Place a flat heavy object such as a large book on your "stomach." Contract your abdominal muscles and lower the object as much as possible. Hold this position for 10 seconds.

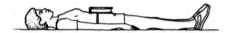

Exercise Six

OBJECTIVE
This is another exercise for strengthening the neck muscles.

DIRECTIONS
Lie on your back on the floor with knees bent and arms crossed over your chest. Place a solid object, three to four inches in height, under your head. Contract your neck muscles and lift your body as high off the floor as you can while keeping your head in contact with the object under it. Hold this position for 10 seconds.

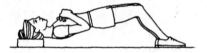

Exercise Seven

OBJECTIVE
This is an additional exercise for strengthening the shoulders, arms, and gluteal region.

DIRECTIONS
Lie on the floor on your back with arms at sides, palms against floor. While keeping your head, hands, and heels in contact with the floor, lift your body as high off the floor as you can. Hold this position for 10 seconds.

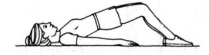

Exercise Eight

OBJECTIVE	This exercise is designed to strengthen the muscles of the hip region.
DIRECTIONS	Lie on the floor on your side with legs extended and feet secured under a low heavy object such as a sofa. Cross arms in front at chest level. Lift the upper trunk as high as possible without bending to the front or back. Hold in this position for 10 seconds.

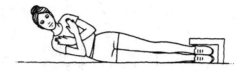

AN ISOTONIC EXERCISE PROGRAM

Isotonic exercises are designed to work on muscle groups, meaning more than one muscle at a time. Therefore it is not necessary, except to avoid boredom, to know a large number of exercises. Ten good exercises performed correctly each day or every other day is sufficient for your exercise program. It is only human to seek variety, but substituting exercises of lesser value will be detrimental to your progress.

The following ten exercises are among the best isotonic exercises and will cover your entire body. Strive to perform each exercise the number of times listed before going on to the next stage. If you find a stage too easy, progress on to the next stage at your next exercise session. Try to perform each movement as accurately as possible and to rest no longer than 1 minute between exercises. Research has shown that it takes at least 20 minutes of continuous exercise to receive maximum benefit from an exercise program.

Continue each stage until you can do the number of repetitions listed, then go on to the next stage. Each stage is progressively more difficult. When you reach the last stage of exercises and can perform all of the repetitions listed, continue the program on a minimum three-day-a-week basis for maintenance purposes.

Remember to use a warm-up and cool-down with each isotonic exercise session. This will help prevent severe muscle soreness.

Push-Ups

BODY AREA Arms, shoulders, chest, and upper back

STAGE ONE *Wall Push-Away* Stand arm's distance away from and facing wall. Feet shoulder-width apart, heels flat on floor. Place palms, fingers up, against the wall at shoulder level. Keep body straight and heels on floor while bending arms until forehead touches wall. Push away from wall back into original position. Begin with 10 repetitions and add 5 repetitions per week.

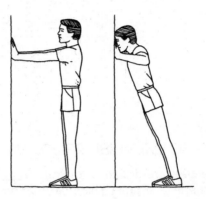

STAGE TWO *Chair Push-Up* Assume incline push-up position with feet on floor and hands on heavy chair or bench, body straight. Place hands shoulder-width apart, fingertips forward, chin up, and chest forward. Lower chest to within two inches of chair and push back up into original position. Begin with 10 repetitions, adding 5 per week.

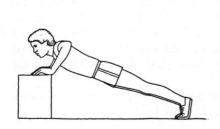
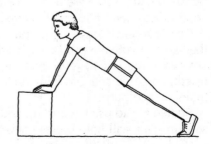

STAGE THREE *Push-Up* Assume a prone position supported by hands and toes, with body and arms straight, hands wide, outside of shoulders, palms flat on floor. Keep chin up and chest forward as you lower chest to within two inches of floor and return to starting position. Repeat 10 times, adding 2 to 5 repetitions per week. Most girls and women will find it difficult to progress from this stage; however, don't be discouraged. You can work into the advanced variations if you want to. It will take more time.

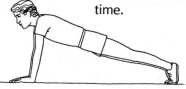

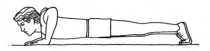

ADVANCED STAGE *Push-Up Variations* Use the same position as in Stage Three but make the following changes:

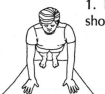

1. Hands shoulder-width apart.

2. Hands narrow, directly underneath breastbone, turned inward with fingertips touching.

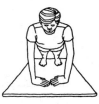

3. Feet elevated on bench and body inclined downward.
4. From hand-stand position with body braced against wall.

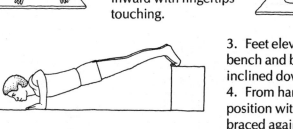

Start with 5 to 10 in each position and work up to 25 repetitions. Continue with 25 in each of the above positions plus 25 of the Stage Three push-up for a total of 100 repetitions.

Boys and men who are interested in body-building and better muscle definition must progress to this level. Use this series of 100 push-ups in your warm-up for weight training lifts.

Chair Rowing[13]

BODY AREA	Upper and center back, shoulders, and chest
STAGE ONE	Place two chairs about five feet apart with backs of chairs facing each other. Place a broomstick across the top of the backs. Lie on floor between chairs and grip the broomstick with hands shoulder-width apart, arms straight. While keeping heels on floor, raise seat until body is straight and supported only by hands and heels. Keeping body straight, pull up to the broomstick until chest touches and return to starting position. If you cannot pull chest all the way up to the broomstick, pull up as far as you can and return to starting position. Keep trying for one perfect repetition. Try to work up to a total of 10 perfect repetitions.

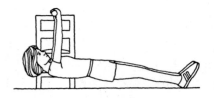

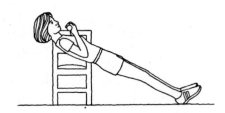

STAGE TWO	Continue same exercise, trying to work up to a total of 25 perfect repetitions.
STAGE THREE	Continue same exercise, trying to work up to a total of 35 perfect repetitions.
ADVANCED STAGE	Continue same exercise. Work up to a total of 50 repetitions.

Broomstick Twist[14]

BODY AREA   Lower back and waistline

STAGE ONE   Use a pole (a cut-off broomstick is excellent) and place it over your shoulders, behind neck, gripping it wide with your hands. Bend forward until your upper body is parallel to the floor while keeping legs straight but not hyperextended. Twist your body in a half-circular motion, bringing the ends of the pole to each foot alternately. Start with a total of 30 repetitions (15 on each side alternately) and work up to a total of 50 (25 on each side).

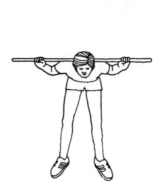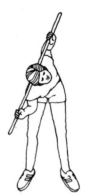

STAGE TWO   Continue same exercise starting with a total of 50 (25 on each side) and work up to a total of 50 on each side for a total of 100 repetitions.

STAGE THREE   Continue same exercise starting with a total of 50 on each side (total of 100) and work up to a total of 75 on each side for a total of 150.

ADVANCED STAGE   Continue same exercise starting with a total of 150 and work up to a total of 200 (100 on each side) or change the pole for a weighted barbell bar with or without weights. Cut repetitions according to the amount of load on the bar. Heavy weights are not recommended for this exercise. They could cause instability.

Side Bend

BODY AREA   Waistline

STAGE ONE   Use the same pole as in the previous exercise. Place on shoulders, behind the neck, while gripping it wide with your hands. Bend from side to side, dropping as far down on each side as possible. Keep the body straight, don't bend backward or forward. Do 25 on each side alternately for a total of 50 repetitions.

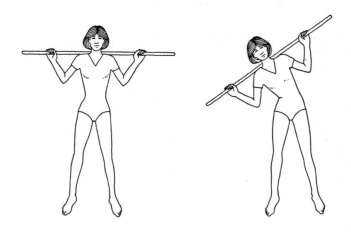

STAGE TWO   Continue same exercise starting with a total of 50 (25 on each side) and work up to a total of 100, 50 on each side.

STAGE THREE   Continue same exercise starting with 50 on each side, for a total of 100; work up to a total of 150, 75 on each side alternately.

ADVANCED STAGE   Continue same exercise starting with a total of 150, (75 on each side) and work up to a total of 200 (100 on each side) or change the pole for a weighted barbell and drop back in repetitions. Heavy weights are not recommended for this exercise. They could cause instability.

Sit-Ups

BODY AREA   Abdominals and lower back

STAGE ONE   Sit on floor, knees bent and feet secured. You may use a heavy object or another person to secure your feet. Cross arms in front of chest and lift head. From this position, roll up to a sitting position and back down. This is one sit-up. Work up to 50 sit-ups.

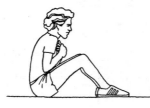 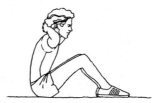

STAGE TWO   Continue same exercise position, with one exception. Change the arms. Place hands behind neck, elbows held back and high. Execute the sit-up in this position. Start with as many as you can do and work up to 75.

STAGE THREE   Continue same position as in Stage Two. Add the twisting sit-up. As you sit up, touch one elbow to the opposite knee and repeat on other side. Work up to 50 regular and 50 twisting for a total of 100.

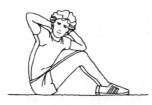 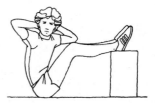

ADVANCED STAGE   To Stage Three add the following isolated sit-up. Place your feet up on the seat of a heavy chair. Sit up from this position. Add 50 in this position to the 100 in Stage Three for a total of 150.

Leg Raises

BODY AREA	Abdominals and lower back
STAGE ONE	Assume a supine (back-lying) position on floor with legs straight and close together, arms at side. While keeping legs straight and together, raise both legs about one foot off the floor and hold for a count of 2, then return to starting position. Start with the number you can do and work up to 25 repetitions.

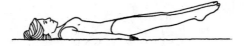

STAGE TWO	Continue same exercise, changing the hold to a count of 5. You might have to drop back in repetitions. Start with as many as you can do and work up to 35 repetitions.
STAGE THREE	Assume supine position, raising legs one foot off floor, then do two leg straddles while keeping legs one foot off floor. Straddle by separating the legs and bringing them back together. Start with as many as you can do and work up to 50 repetitions.

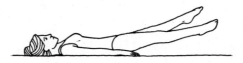

ADVANCED STAGE	Continue same exercise, changing to five leg straddles before returning legs to floor. Work up to 50 repetitions.

Supine Lifts

BODY AREA	Gluteals (seat), hips, and thighs
STAGE ONE	Assume a sitting crab position with hands on floor behind you, fingertips forward, knees bent. Raise the body, belly to the ceiling, so that it is parallel to the floor and supported only by the hands and feet. Return to the starting position. Start with 15 and work up to 25 repetitions.

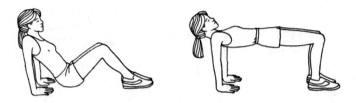

STAGE TWO	Continue same exercise and work up to 50 repetitions.
STAGE THREE	Use the sitting crab position, but this time as you lift your seat, extend one leg. Return to the starting position and repeat, lifting opposite leg. Work up to 50 on each leg alternately for a total of 100.

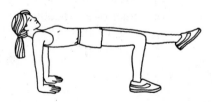

ADVANCED STAGE	Use the sitting crab position. Lift the seat until body is parallel to the floor, then extend each leg alternately five times before returning to the starting position. Work up to 50 repetitions with 5 leg lifts on each leg during each repetition.

Half Squats

BODY AREA   Gluteals, hips, and thighs

STAGE ONE   Assume a standing position with body straight and feet no more than one foot apart. Keeping body straight, bend knees and lower seat (squat) halfway to floor so that the seat is parallel to floor. Hold this position (1) for a count of 5. Work up to 25 repetitions.

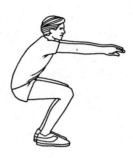

STAGE TWO   Continue doing 25 repetitions of the previous exercise and add 25 repetitions of position 2: use the same exercise but widen the stance. Stand with feet three feet apart as you do the same exercise. You should work up to 25 repetitions in position 1 and 25 repetitions in position 2 for a total of 50 repetitions.

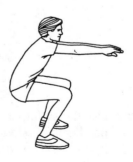

STAGE THREE   Add position 3: after assuming the squat position 1, while remaining in the squat position take five steps forward and five steps backward, then return to the starting position. Work up to 25 repetitions. Added to position 1 and 2, this will be a total of 75 repetitions.

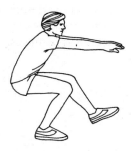

ADVANCED STAGE   Assume the half-squat position with legs almost together. While remaining in that position, jump five times, and come back to the same position each time. Then return to the starting position and repeat 25 times. Add to positions 1, 2, and 3 for a total of 100 repetitions.

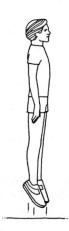

Heel Raises

BODY AREA   Ankles and calves

STAGE ONE   Stand on book or other 3- to 6-inch object with heels resting off edge of object on floor. From this position, with arms raised at sides for balance, raise all of the way up onto the toes and return to starting position. Work up to 25 repetitions.

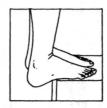

STAGE TWO   To the 25 repetitions with feet parallel, add 25 repetitions with feet turned in for a total of 50 repetitions.

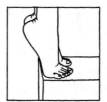

STAGE THREE   Add to the previous positions 25 repetitions with the feet turned out for a total of 75 repetitions.

ADVANCED STAGE Work up to 50 repetitions in each of the three positions for a total of 150 repetitions.

EXERCISES FOR ANKLES AND CALVES

Jumps in Place

BODY AREA Ankles and calves

STAGE ONE With feet parallel and about one foot apart, jump in place 25 times while keeping a steady pace.

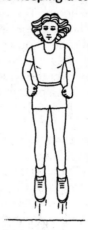

STAGE TWO Add 25 jumps on the right foot and 25 jumps on the left foot to the previous, for a total of 75 repetitions.

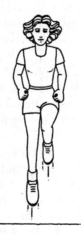

STAGE THREE Add 25 jumps with feet apart for a total of 100 repetitions.

ADVANCED STAGE Work toward repeating the entire series 5 times.

WEIGHT TRAINING

Weight training is one of the most efficient and effective ways to develop strength, contour the female figure, and give better shape, size, and muscle definition to the male build. Persons of all ages, both male and female, use weight training as a form of exercise to keep in shape. These same persons spend millions of dollars each year to join health clubs and spas where they can use weight training equipment. Many who do not join have basic weight training equipment at home. The number of persons purchasing weight-training machines for home use is increasing yearly. In fact, major department stores and mail-order houses are producing small weight-training machines and barbell sets on an assembly-line basis. Most important, coaches and trainers all over the country are finally advocating weight training as a means of improving performance and preventing and rehabilitating injuries.[15]

BACKGROUND   Some years ago, weight training was confined mostly to body builders and competitive weight lifters. However, owing to the efforts of an Army surgeon, Thomas L. DeLorme, the concept of using weight training to develop strength in the average person and athlete was established during the 1940s. Dr. DeLorme, who was a body builder himself, published a program called Progressive Resistance Exercise in 1951.[16] His concepts provide the basis for weight training as we know it today.

Many misconceptions about weight training existed in the past. It was thought to produce the "muscle-bound" individual, to cause a person to become inflexible, to reduce one's speed, and to cause women to become masculine looking. Research has disproved these old theories, and we now know the benefits of such exercise for both men and women.

BASIC WEIGHT TRAINING   Weight training is too complex and detailed to be covered thoroughly in a general exercise book of this sort. However, the following information is provided in order to get you started and to prepare you for more advanced training if you want it. There may be many times when you will find yourself in situations where you can take part in a weight-training program if you know basically what to do.

It is important to use excellent posture whether sitting, standing, or lying down. Keep your back straight at all times, never let it sway—and that goes for when you are lying on a bench as well. For instance, in exercises where you are lying on your back on the bench, lift your head and feet as this illustration suggests. This will keep your back straight and flat. In standing exercises, keep your legs straight with knees loose. Don't hyperextend the knees, because this can injure them. Never strain with a weight. Use a

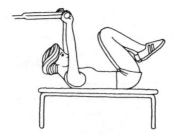

spotter (someone to help you) or a rack, sometimes called a squat rack. Never attempt heavy lifting without a spotter.

It is important to move the weight along the full range of motion, from complete extension of a joint to complete contraction of a muscle on every repetition.[17]

The rest between repetitions and sets varies depending on the weight you are lifting and the type of program. Unless you are on a heavy-load program, working five or six days a week, you should rest for 30 seconds to 1 minute between sets and exercises. Persons on heavy training programs should rest 3 to 5 minutes between sets and exercises.[18]

Breathing theories vary, and there are almost as many theories as there are experts in weightlifting. Concentrating on a breathing technique seems to be of major importance only to the heavy lifter. In this case, the most common technique is to exhale on the resistance phase of the lift and inhale on the recovery phase. For instance, when doing a push-up, exhale as you push your body up and inhale as you lower it.[19] In a lift, exhale as you lift the weight, expelling all breath at the top of the lift. Inhale as you lower the weight. Remember, breathing theories *are* contradictory, and if the above technique seems very awkward, you are probably not lifting a heavy enough load to warrant concentration on breathing.

Check the equipment before each lift. Make certain that pins in machine weights are secure, and that pulleys and cables are on track. Check collars and plates on free weights. If the collars are not secure, the plate will slip off the bar. Check all bolts and screws for tightness. If this seems time-consuming, remember that injuries are more time-consuming, and hurt besides.

Warm up before lifting, always. Refer to the information on warming up in Chapter 5. Muscle cramps can occur if the muscles are not ready for exercise.

Flexibility exercise is of major importance to individuals who are weightlifting. The flexibility program can act as a cool-down—that is, when you perform flexibility exercises after a weight-training workout. Whether you use flexibility exercises as a finish to your weight training workout or as an alternate-day program, be certain to include them.

Sets and repetitions vary according to the lifter's goals. A repetition is one execution of an exercise; ten push-ups are ten repetitions. A set is a grouping of repetitions; thus two sets of eight repetitions would be sixteen repetitions done in groups of eight with rest in between. If maximum muscular *strength* is desired, the training program will emphasize greater resistance (weight or load) with fewer repetitions; if maximum muscular *endurance* is desired, the program will emphasize many repetitions against less resistance.[20]

TWO WEIGHT-TRAINING PROGRAMS

The following programs are designed to develop an even balance of muscular strength and muscular endurance. They are for both men and women, and will satisfy the beginning to intermediate lifter. For more advanced information and more varied techniques, consult the notes to this chapter.

The exercises will be explained by illustration only at the end of the chapter. Most gyms and clubs, and even weight-training sets that you can buy, provide written instruction as well as picture illustrations of weight-training exercises. Please understand also that there are many more exercises than it is possible to describe and illustrate in this book.

To begin you must first establish the amount of load to use for each exercise. Through trial and error find the amount of weight that will just barely allow you to finish each set. If you can finish the number of repetitions in each set easily, then your load is too light, and you should increase it at the next exercise session. *Remember to do all of the sets of each exercise consecutively before going on to the next exercise.* You will know that your load is too heavy if you cannot finish all of the sets of an exercise. If this happens, decrease the load at the next exercise session.

Progression is accomplished by doing one or a combination of the following:

1. Increase the load of an exercise when all sets become easy to perform.
2. Add another set when all sets of an exercise become easy to perform. This progression must be used when your weight sets can no longer increase in load, as they should do.
3. Change your set and repetitions system.
4. Add workout sessions.

The above methods are based on the principle that in order to make progress, you must increase the intensity, duration, or frequency of an exercise or exercise sessions. The programs given here are designed to help you make that progression.

A three-day and six-day program are shown. You must choose the one that best fits your time schedule. Keep in mind that the six-day program will allow faster progression. Also, the six-day program is divided into upper and lower body phases, so that your muscles will receive the one day of needed rest between lifting sessions.

Three-Day Program

Begin with one set of twelve repetitions. Every two weeks add one set and decrease the repetitions by two:

Weeks 1 and 2:	1 set of 12 reps
Weeks 3 and 4:	2 sets of 10 reps
Weeks 4 and 5:	3 sets of 8 reps

When you reach the sixth week, continue the 3 sets of 8 reps but before doing them add 1 set of 12 reps as follows:

Weeks 6 and 7:	1 set of 12 reps
	3 sets of 8 reps
Weeks 8 and 9:	2 sets of 12 reps
	3 sets of 8 reps

On the tenth and eleventh weeks, continue this program and add to the end of it 2 sets of 4 reps. Your program from now on will be as follows, except where a change is noted:

2 sets of 12 reps
3 sets of 8 reps.
2 sets of 4 reps

EXERCISES

1. Incline Sit-Up: 1 set of 25 reps only
2. Leg-Overs: 1 set of 25 reps only
3. Bench Press
4. Leg Press
5. Shoulder Press
6. Leg Extension
7. Lat Pulldown
8. Leg Curl or Hack Lift
9. Upright Rowing
10. Heel Raises or Toe Press
11. Dumbbell Flyes: 1 set of 25 reps

12. Dumbbell Pullover: 1 set of 25 reps
13. Dumbbell Curls: 1 set of 25 reps, each arm, alternately
14. Bench Press or Triceps Extension: 1 set of 25 reps

Six-Day Program

Days 1, 3, and 5

Except where indicated, use the following set system:

> 2 sets of 12 reps
> 2 sets of 8 reps
> 2 sets of 6 reps

EXERCISES

1. Push-ups: 1 set of 25 reps
2. Chin-ups: 1 set of 25 reps
3. Bench Press
4. Lat Pulldown
5. Shoulder Press (military)
6. Upright Rowing
7. Triceps Extension (French press)
8. Regular Grip Dumbbell Curl: 1 set of 25 reps each arm, alternate
9. Reverse Grip Dumbbell Curl: 1 set of 25 reps each arm, alternate
10. Bent-arm Pullover: 1 set of 25 reps
11. Bent-arm Lateral Raise (flyes): 1 set of 25 reps
12. Wrist Curl: 1 set of 25 reps with regular grip, 1 set of 25 reps with reverse grip

Days 2, 4, and 6

Except where indicated, use the following set system:

> 2 sets of 12 reps
> 2 sets of 8 reps
> 2 sets of 4 reps

EXERCISES

1. Sit-Ups (incline): 1 set of 25 reps
2. Leg-Overs: 1 set of 25 reps
3. Leg Raises: 1 set of 25 reps
4. Leg Press or Half-Squat
5. Leg Extension

6. Leg Curl or Hack Lift
7. Toe Press or Heel Raises
8. Deadlift
9. Forward Bend (Good Morning): 1 set of 25 reps
10. Waist Twist: 1 set of 25 reps, alternate each side
11. Side Bend: 1 set of 25 reps, alternate each side
12. Side Leg: Lifts (pulley or ankle weight): 1 set of 25 reps each side

RECORDING YOUR EXERCISES

Appendix D contains Weight-Training Record Sheets on which you can record your weight-training exercises. It is important for you to keep a record of the load used for each set of each exercise. Here is an example of how to record an exercise. The number of repetitions is recorded in the upper left

Date	3/10			3/12			3/14			3/16		
3. *Bench Press*	12/90	12/90	8/100	12/90	12/90	8/110	12/100	12/100	8/110	12/100	12/100	8/110
	8/100	6/110	6/110	8/110	6/110	6/110	8/110	6/110	6/110	8/110	6/120	6/120

half of the square, and the weight lifted that day is recorded in the lower right half. If you cannot complete the number of sets listed, leave the square blank. As you are able to complete the number of sets and repetitions, record them in the appropriate squares for that day's workout and move upward in load.

EQUIPMENT

The exercises in your program are designed to use both free and machine weights. If one or the other, or a substitute, is not available, you will have to eliminate the exercise. There are enough exercises in both programs to enable you to eliminate one or two without drastically slowing your progress.

Here is a word especially for women: sometimes you will find machine weights too heavy for you. If this is the case, begin with a free weight, such as a dumbbell or barbell, and work up to the point where you can use the machine weights.

If you want to set up your own exercise studio at home, you can buy free-weight equipment at reasonable prices. Even a few small machines are available at a reasonable price. However, such purchases can quickly add up to a lot of money. With the increasing number of health spas and athletic clubs available today, it would be wise to inquire about their membership fees. Joining a club might be less expensive than buying your own equipment. Also, if something prevents you from following this form of exercise, you have not spent needlessly.

The equipment you will need is indicated for each exercise. In some cases, the exercise can be performed on both machines and with free weights.

CLOTHING

Wear clothes that are comfortable and will not restrict movement: a warm-up outfit (either a jogging suit or sweatshirt and loose long pants), shorts, leotards, socks, and tennis shoes or athletic shoes. It is important that men wear supporters and women wear bras; such support is necessary during weight training for safety's sake. Women might want to purchase golf gloves with the fingers cut out for both hands (weight-training gloves are usually much too large for women). These will help prevent callouses from forming on the palms of the hands. They will also help your grip. A weight-training midsection support belt is also necessary for heavy lifters. These are available in most clubs and can also be purchased in sporting goods stores. Be sure to buy the correct size for you.

A FINAL WORD

Before you begin your program, keep this in mind: there will be times when you do not seem to progress, times when you will hit a plateau. When this happens, take a week off from training. Don't do any deliberate exercise during this week off. Let it be a mental as well as a physical rest from exercise. Then resume your program where you left off. Many people have found success with this technique. Your weeks of rest should not occur too frequently, however; if you lay off more often than one week out of every three months, this technique is unlikely to work.

WEIGHT-TRAINING EXERCISES

The weight-training exercises that follow can be used in the three-day and six-day programs described previously. Although each program covers the entire body, the exercises show more specifically the body areas that will be benefited. The illustrations provided will enable you to perform the exercises properly.

WEIGHT-TRAINING EXERCISES

Push-Up

BODY AREA   Chest, shoulders, and back of upper arm

EQUIPMENT   None

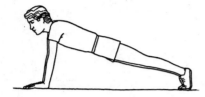

Chin-Up

BODY AREA   Shoulders, upper back, biceps area of upper arm, lower arm

EQUIPMENT   Overhead chinning bar

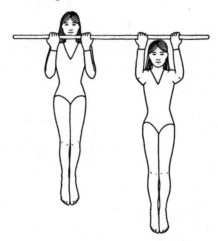

Bench Press

BODY AREA   Shoulders, chest, and back of upper arm

EQUIPMENT   Machine, or bench and barbell

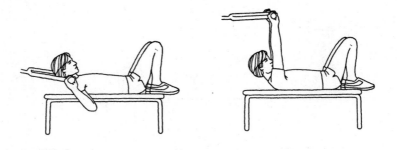

Lat Pulldown

BODY AREA   Shoulders, upper back, chest, and back of upper arm

EQUIPMENT   Machine

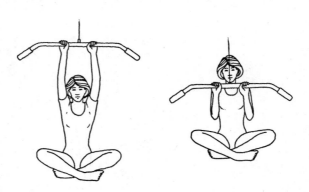

Shoulder Press

BODY AREA   Shoulder and upper arm

EQUIPMENT   Machine or barbell

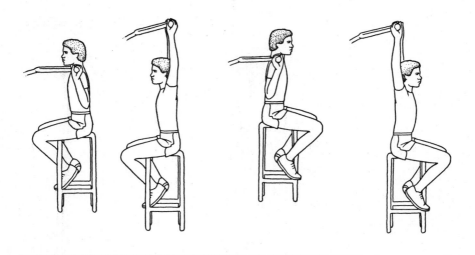

Upright Rowing

BODY AREA   Shoulders, upper arm, lower arm

EQUIPMENT   Machine or barbell

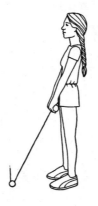 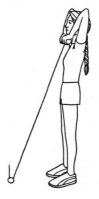

Triceps Extension

BODY AREA   Shoulders, back of upper arm

EQUIPMENT   Machine or barbell

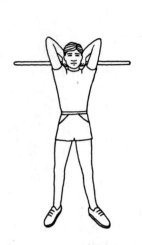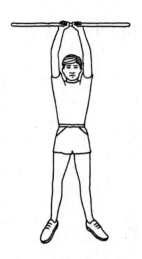

Dumbbell Curl

BODY AREA   Lower arm

EQUIPMENT   Dumbbells (can also be performed with a barbell as shown; do 25 reps)

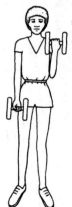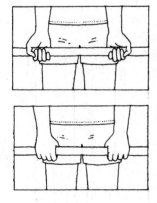

Bent-Arm Pullover

BODY AREA   Chest and shoulders

EQUIPMENT   Barbell, dumbbell, or plate

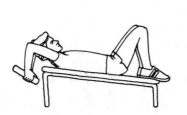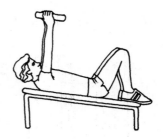

Lateral Raise (Flyes)

BODY AREA   Chest and shoulders

EQUIPMENT   Dumbbells or plate

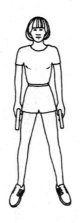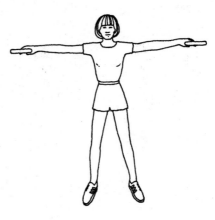

Wrist Curls

BODY AREA   Lower arms and wrists

EQUIPMENT   Barbell or dumbbells

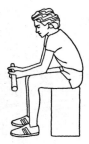 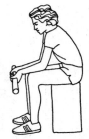 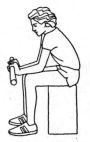 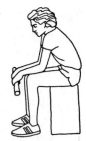

Sit-Ups

BODY AREA   Abdominals and lower back

EQUIPMENT   Incline board

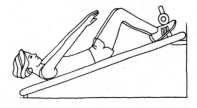 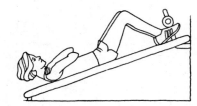

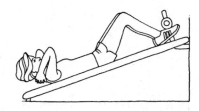

Leg-Overs

BODY AREA   Abdominals and lower back

EQUIPMENT   Incline board

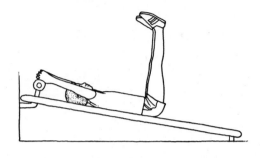

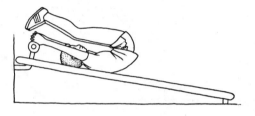

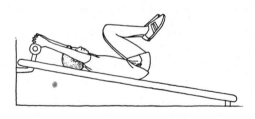

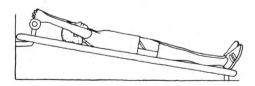

Leg Raises

BODY AREA   Abdominals and lower back

EQUIPMENT   Incline board or floor

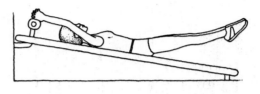

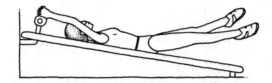

Leg Press or Half Squat

BODY AREA   Buttocks, lower back, and thighs

EQUIPMENT   Machine, or barbell

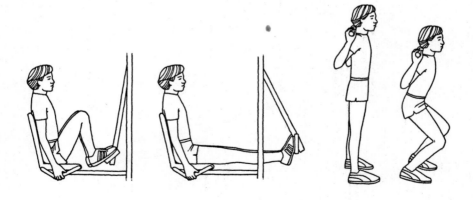

Leg Extension

BODY AREA	Anterior thighs or quadriceps
EQUIPMENT	Machine

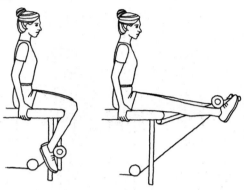

Leg Curl or Hack Lift

BODY AREA	Posterior thighs or hamstrings
EQUIPMENT	Machine or barbell

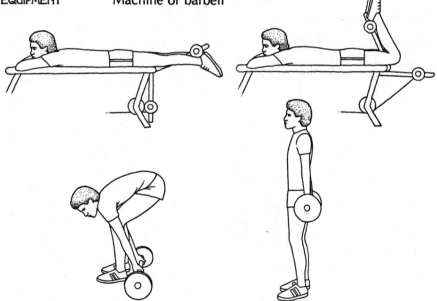

Toe Press or Heel Raise

BODY AREA   Lower leg (calf)

EQUIPMENT   Machine or barbell

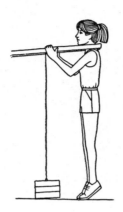
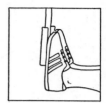
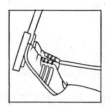

Deadlift (straight leg, or bent knee)

BODY AREA   Lower back, hamstrings, buttocks

EQUIPMENT   Barbell

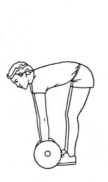
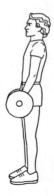
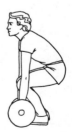

Forward Bend

BODY AREA   Lower back, anterior and posterior thighs

EQUIPMENT   Barbell

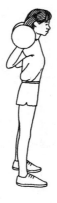
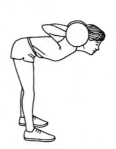

Waist Twist

BODY AREA   Waistline

EQUIPMENT   Barbell

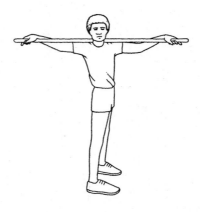

Side Bend

BODY AREA   Waistline

EQUIPMENT   Barbell

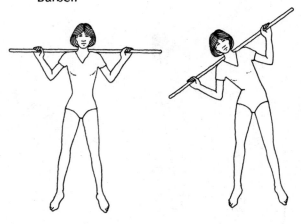

Side Leg Lifts

BODY AREA   Buttocks and thighs

EQUIPMENT   Pulley, machine, or ankle weights

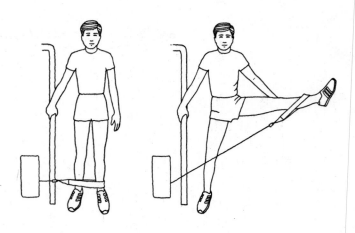

Notes

1. William J. Stone and William A. Kroll, *Sports Conditioning and Weight Training* (Boston: Allyn and Bacon, Inc., 1978), p. 6.

2. *Ibid.,* p. 38.

3. Herbert A. deVries, *Physiology of Exercise* (Dubuque: Wm. C. Brown Company Publishers, 1974), p. 229.

4. Peter V. Karpovich and Wayne E. Sinning, *Physiology of Muscular Activity* (Philadelphia: W. B. Saunders Company, 1971), pp. 26–27.

5. DeVries, *Physiology of Exercise,* p. 379.

6. Harold B. Falls, Earl L. Wallis, and Gene A. Logan, *Foundations of Conditioning* (New York: Academic Press, 1970), pp. 76–77.

7. Anthony A. Annarino, *Developmental Conditioning for Physical Education and Athletics* (St. Louis: The C. V. Mosby Company, 1976), p. 81.

8. *Ibid.,* p. 1.

9. Jack H. Wilmore, *Athletic Training and Physical Fitness* (Boston: Allyn and Bacon, Inc., 1977), p. 68.

10. Frank Vitale, *Individualized Fitness Programs* (Englewood Cliffs: Prentice-Hall, Inc., 1973), pp. 122–23.

11. Gene Hooks, *Weight Training in Athletics and Physical Education* (Englewood Cliffs: Prentice-Hall, Inc., 1974), p. 17.

12. *Ibid.,* p. 23.

13. Arnold Schwarzenegger and Douglas Kent Hall, *Arnold: The Education of A Bodybuilder* (New York: Pocket Books, 1977), p. 166.

14. *Ibid.,* p. 169.

15. Ellington Darden, "Winning with Strength," *Athletic Purchasing and Facilities* (January 1979), p. 31.

16. Phillip J. Rasch, *Weight Training* (Dubuque: Wm. C. Brown Company Publishers, 1975), p. 1.

17. Bill Reynolds, *Complete Weight Training Book* (Mountain View: World Publications, 1976), p. 35.

18. Stone and Kroll, *Sports Conditioning,* p. 38

19. Schwarzenegger and Hall, *Education of a Body Builder,* p. 162.

20. Stone and Kroll, p. 37.

9 | *CREATING A MORE ACTIVE ENVIRONMENT*

In the most rapidly changing environment to which man has ever been exposed, we remain pitifully ignorant of how the human animal copes.

ALVIN TOFFLER
Future Shock

Though many persons have found the knack of changing their lifestyle, too few of us recognize that there are specific skills involved, or even that we have control over our ability to adapt creatively to our environment. From the previous chapters, we realize that we are the victims, as well as the perpetrators, of our automated society. We are also aware of the results of sedentary behavior, such as sitting and reclining for periods of time. Even thirty minutes of such inactivity can decrease the blood flow to the brain, resulting in sluggishness.[1]

Yet it seems that we go out of our way to be sedentary and actually seek out sedentary activities. In order to counteract this tendency, we must reorganize our environment to provide maximum activity and readjust our lifestyle to it.

CHANGING THE HOME ENVIRONMENT

Changing our movement habits is not as difficult as it might seem if we consider the ways in which we meet the demands of our daily activities. For example, we can move the telephone so that we must walk a few steps to use it and must stand up while using it. Remember, even standing still uses more calories than sitting. Or we can place frequently used items such as books, clothes, or canned goods on the high shelves, where we must stretch

115

in order to reach them. A careful look at your home and work area will bring to mind many more examples.

The performance of many daily chores can be modified to increase strength and flexibility. For example, carry grocery sacks in your arms or in a cart and walk instead of using the car; stand while putting on your shoes and socks or stockings; climb stairs whenever possible; pump your own gas and wash your windshield while you are at it; and sweep the driveway instead of washing it down with a hose. You can incorporate fitness exercises into your daily habits, and at the same time conserve the nation's energy. To increase your desire to change, remind yourself that washing your·own car and mowing your own lawn are investments in health as well as money-saving practices. Moving furniture when cleaning house will contribute to muscular strength as well as a better cleaning job.

If you will honestly admit the importance of exercise, it will be easy to find the time and the place. It's simply a matter of priorities.

—DONALD VICKERY
Life Plan for Your Health

Take a moment and mentally go through your normal day, concentrating on those habits that could be modified. As an example, mid-morning and mid-afternoon periods are often interrupted by "breaks," which are usually spent sitting and eating. Instead, try a "walk-break." This will provide physical exercise and decrease the number of calories you take in.

EXERCISE AT WORK

Walk-breaks can be done at work, too. How many times do you find yourself riding the elevator instead of walking the stairs? One executive we know climbs the fourteen flights of stairs to his office each day as a part of his exercise program. Many persons now ride bicycles to work and use their lunch breaks to go down to a gym for almost an hour of exercise (eating a light lunch afterwards). A good breakfast and a mid-morning snack as well can easily compensate for missing the noontime meal. One woman we know walks the hall outside her office. She uses a pedometer to record the mileage and makes a point of walking two miles per day.

You do not have to change into exercise clothes to do many exercises. You can close your office door and do sit-ups, push-ups, and stretching exercises. You will find that the increased circulation caused by this movement will make you feel more energetic. Through conscious application, you should be able to change many things at work that will make your workday more active.

PROVIDING YOUR OWN EXERCISE EQUIPMENT

Besides incorporating fitness habits into our daily schedule, we must also set aside time for regular exercise, either in our own home or in a gym designed for that purpose. Many persons provide for exercise right in their own home, sometimes quite elaborately. Many media stars keep in shape at home on Universal's Centurion, a superdeluxe, $4,000 weight-training machine. Marcy Gymnasium Equipment's Family Fitness Center, which costs $1,500, provides exercise for others.[2]

However, exercise equipment does not have to be expensive. Without realizing it, you probably have available the materials necessary for beginning a weight-training program like the one presented in Chapter 8. Among the many household items that can be used for weights are these:

Weight	Items
1 lb.	Cans of fruit or vegetables (labels always list weight)
2 lbs.	Quart of water in plastic bottle (use juice or liquid detergent bottles) Large cans of vegetables
3 lbs.	48 oz. bottle of water Electric iron
4–5 lbs.	2 quart plastic bottle of water (use one that is easy to grip) 6½ cups of sand in a 56 oz. bottle
8–10 lbs.	A one-gallon plastic bottle filled with sand or water

If you look around the house or garage, you will probably find many more items you can use.

However, if you prefer "pumping iron" instead of plastic, weight-training sets can be purchased inexpensively. Try the discount department stores, sporting goods stores, and even equipment swaps. You should be able to buy a bar with assorted weights and a set of dumbbells with assorted weights for under fifty dollars.

You will need one long bar (five to six feet in length); two short, dumbbell bars; collars and pins to secure the weights; and an assortment of weight plates ranging from 2.5 to 25 pounds each. There are two kinds of weight plates, vinyl-covered cement and cast iron. The vinyl-covered cement plates are the least expensive, but they can break if dropped, whereas cast-iron plates are very nearly indestructible. The Olympic weight sets are expensive, but they are a good investment if you expect to continue a weight-training program for some time.

If you are serious about making weight training a part of your exercise program, and you can afford it, you may want to invest in a home gym such as the ones mentioned previously. These are available through various department and sporting goods stores, as well as through their own distributors. There are many different kinds, so you will want to do some investigating before you purchase one. Be sure that it will meet all your needs.

Such machines can often be purchased on an installment-payment plan. Although a machine is far more expensive than a free-weight set, its versatility and efficiency may outweigh the increased cost over a few years.

JOINING A HEALTH CLUB OR SPA

A recommended alternative to purchasing your own equipment is to purchase a health club membership. Maybe your career requires you to travel or relocate frequently. Perhaps your home is not large enough for weight equipment, and adding a room would cost you thousands of dollars. Or perhaps exercising with a group appeals to you. In these and many other cases, membership in a health club or spa is the alternative.

These clubs usually provide a weight-training room, an exercise floor, a jogging track, a swimming pool, a jacuzzi, a steam room, and a sauna. Some clubs also have racquet ball and tennis courts available, in most cases, for additional fees. The cost usually includes a one-time initiation fee and a

---

There are more than 3000 health spas around the nation, ranging from small exercise rooms and reducing salons to multimillion dollar facilities with gymnasiums, swimming pools, running tracks, saunas, whirlpools, and the like.

— CONSUMER REPORTS
August 1978

---

monthly charge. Some clubs operate on a monthly charge only or a yearly charge only. A very few offer a share-type membership which may be sold if the owner wishes to discontinue membership. The cost of various memberships ranges from $50 to over $5,000 per year.

When choosing a club, make certain that it hires experienced, knowledgeable personnel; that its equipment is adequate; and that its open hours will serve your needs.

> The Federal Trade Commission says it has received "a substantial number of complaints" from consumers who charge they are victimized by bait-and-switch advertising and offers of fictitious bargains, by misrepresentation of facilities and personnel, and by misleading explanations about contracts.
>
> — CONSUMER REPORTS
> August 1978

Consumers Union, one of three organizations designated by the Federal Trade Commission to investigate health spas, recommends that you ask the following questions before joining:

1. Does the spa try to sell long-term contracts on the first visit, promising a special reduced rate?

2. Can you sign up for a short-term program and try the spa for a few weeks, or pay by the visit for a trial period?

3. Will the spa provide a written guarantee of a "cooling-off" period with a fair refund policy?

4. Does the spa take a medical history and suggest you see a doctor before starting a program? Consumers Union concludes with this warning: "No matter what the other qualities of the spa, if it ignores medical histories, the personnel aren't adequately trained."[3]

TAKING ADVANTAGE OF COMMUNITY AGENCIES

A less expensive alternative to commercial clubs and spas can be found in most communities. Local YMCAs and YWCAs offer various exercise programs and facilities, managed and staffed by experienced personnel. Many high schools and colleges provide a variety of programs offered through their community-service or adult-education departments. Community recreation agencies also offer many type of physical fitness programs. You will be certain of receiving quality instruction through any one of these agencies.

The cost of these programs is usually low—in most cases, not over a hundred dollars a year.

EQUIPMENT AND FADS TO AVOID

Machines that roll, shake, or jiggle are not only worthless, but in many cases injurious.[4] These machines can stretch the skin, leaving stretch marks and bruises, and in some cases they have even caused abrasions. Body wraps are also ineffective. The weight lost through perspiration will always be regained upon consuming liquids, and extreme water losses can be dangerous. The same principle goes for rubberized warm-up suits and waist and thigh belts. Though all these can be dangerous, the rubberized warm-up suit is the most dangerous because of its coverage. Don't waste your money or jeopardize your health by using these devices.

A great amount of money is earned by unscrupulous vendors who advertise devices that are supposed to create a beautiful figure or muscular build; or pills and formulas supposed to help one lose weight fast; and books and devices purported to make one instantly healthier. Among the thousands of methods there are a few that really work; most, however, are false and inaccurate. The methods that really do work are also the ones that require more energy from us, which is why they are sometimes not the most popular.

If we do not believe in magic, why do we—the American people—spend hard-earned money on "magic formulas" for losing weight, staying young, or improving our looks? One reason is the media blitz directed at us. We are bombarded by advertisements on television and radio, in magazines and newspapers. We are the only ones who can end this; we can refuse to be fooled or to make foolish purchases by learning more about our bodies, about nutrition, and about exercise.

EXERCISE CAUTIONS

A few common exercises can be more damaging than beneficial, especially to persons with weak muscles in the area being affected. The following exercises fit into this category:

1. Double leg lifts, double leg raises, straight-leg sit-ups, and jackknife sit-ups should not be attempted by beginners, by persons with weak backs or abdominal muscles, or by persons with a tilted pelvis (swayback).
2. Extreme back bends or any position that tilts the abdomen forward, thus stretching the abdominal muscles, should be attempted only by people with strong abdominal muscles and with no signs of swayback.

3. Deep-knee bends or squats can stretch the knee ligaments and/or pinch the lubricating membrane of the joint and are considered injurious. However, half-knee bends are acceptable when the feet are positioned directly under the knees. This position prevents any twisting motion to the joint.[5]

One should be careful when trying any new exercise position. A good rule is this: if the exercise causes you to strain severely, or if it causes real pain rather than moderate discomfort, eliminate it. Exercises sometimes cause temporary discomfort, but they should never cause severe pain.

EXERCISE WHEN TRAVELING

Travel is the age-old excuse for gaining weight. "But I was on vacation and traveling—how could I exercise?" Well, our bodies and minds can use a vacation from work, but never from our fitness program. Strength, endurance, and flexibility decrease significantly with each inactive day. Therefore, before you travel, it is important to plan for exercise as carefully as you plan for other aspects of your trip.

Most hotel and motel rooms provide enough space for you to do your flexibility and strength exercises. Endurance exercise may be accomplished by running in place, running the stairs, or running in the parking lot. If there is a swimming pool, that's an added advantage. Some hotels and motels now provide a special exercise room.

On a long automobile trip, stop occasionally and run ten times around your car. It may look strange, but works wonders. You might also want to take your tennis racket with you, so you can stop at a school or park along the way for a game of tennis. If you plan for it, you can make your vacation healthful as well as relaxing. All it takes is a little extra thought before you leave.

THE PAR COURSE OR "FITNESSBAHN"

These "planned exercise courses," which originated in Switzerland and Germany, are now increasing in popularity in the United States. They consist of a planned jogging route with various stops along the way where prescribed strength and flexibility exercises are performed. A good course contains a complete exercise program and directs you along its way by signs. If you follow the directions, you can use a par course for your complete exercise program. In addition to providing for complete physical fitness, they offer it in a natural setting.

EXERCISE THROUGH SPORTS AND GAMES

Sports and games, although often excellent for using up calories and for providing fitness exercise for certain areas of the body, are not all equal in fitness value and no one of them will promote all aspects of physical fitness. Table 8, prepared by the President's Council on Physical Fitness, rates the benefits of selected activities on a scale of 0 to 3 points. A team of seven medical experts rated the contribution of each activity to each component. A score of 21 on any component means that all seven experts gave the sport or activity the maximum of 3 points in that area.

> The sharp growth in sports participation can be attributed to such significant factors as increased leisure time, growing affluence, emphases on the importance of physical fitness, and television coverage of sports events.
>
> —DONALD WEISKOPF
> A Guide to Recreation and Leisure

The biggest advantage of sports and games is that they get you out of your chair or away from the TV set. They make you move and therefore make you burn off more calories and spend less time eating. Another advantage of sports and games can be the competitive factor offered. Enjoyable competition allows us to release physical and emotional tension, which can help us to tolerate increased stress in our daily lives.

EXERCISE AND AGING

The need for exercise continues throughout our lives. Population trends for the United States indicate that we are rapidly becoming a nation of older people.[6] Many physical differences exist between individuals, but in one way we are all alike—we all grow older every year, and although no one can completely escape the physical effects of aging, research suggests that exercise and conditioning may slow down the aging processes that curtail physical functioning.[7]

MUSCULAR STRENGTH   We know that muscular strength reaches a peak in the middle to late twenties and begins a gradual decline thereafter. If physical activity levels remain constant, muscle mass will remain relatively stable through the thirties and into the forties.[8] Although much more research needs to be done, we can assume that regular conditioning in our early years

TABLE 8 Fitness Benefits of Various Sports and Games

Activity	Stamina	Muscular endurance	Muscular strength	Flexibility	Total
Swimming	21	20	14	15	70
Handball or squash	19	18	15	16	68
Skiing, cross-country	19	19	15	14	67
Jogging	21	20	17	9	67
Basketball	19	17	15	13	64
Skiing, downhill	16	18	15	14	63
Skating, ice or roller	18	17	15	13	63
Bicycling	19	18	16	9	62
Tennis	16	16	14	14	60
Calisthenics	10	13	16	19	58
Walking	13	14	11	7	45
Golf, using cart	8	8	9	8	33
Bowling	5	5	5	7	22

SOURCE: President's Council on Physical Fitness, *How Different Sports Rate in Promoting Physical Fitness*, U.S. Department of Health, Education and Welfare, No. 253-659 (1978) pp. 4–5.

will help us reach a higher peak of muscular strength, so that our gradual decline will start from a higher point.

THE CARDIOVASCULAR AND RESPIRATORY SYSTEMS Research suggests that cardiovascular and respiratory endurance declines more rapidly than muscular strength.[9] The effects of endurance conditioning upon aging are not scientifically proved as yet, but recent research on elderly marathon runners suggests that such conditioning does help prolong the function of the cardiovascular and respiratory systems.

FLEXIBILITY A decreased range of motion may, more than any other factor, cause a person to feel old. (A twenty-year-old may feel fifty for a short time after a month in a hospital bed.) It seems that only continuous regular exercise can constantly guard against decreasing flexibility, which may be the most difficult component of muscular efficiency to regain once it is allowed to degenerate.[10] According to Laurence Morehouse, who has done extensive research in the field of gerontology, physical age has a variable of thirty years.[11] It is possible, in other words, to be fifty years in chronological age and yet only thirty years or so in physical body age. In a sense, you are only as old as you feel and function. If your conditioning allows you to maintain a full range of motion, you will probably feel much younger than you are.

EMOTIONAL CONSIDERATIONS   "People who continue to be involved in useful activity are more likely to enjoy long, enjoyable lives than are those who 'drop out.' "[12] "One can be chronologically old and think or act young, by associating with newness and innovation in order to remain youthfully vigorous in thought."[13] Our emotions are directly affected by how we feel, and we usually feel better when we are physically active.

TIPS FOR BEGINNERS OVER THIRTY   Degeneration occurs when something is not used. Although it is not possible to stop the final effects of aging, it is possible to delay many effects of the aging process. Persons who maintain physical activity throughout their lives retain a higher degree of strength, flexibility, and endurance or cardiac output than those who live relatively inactive lives.[14]

Old and young alike will benefit from the same type of exercise programs. Older persons, however, should progress more slowly in the early stages of a conditioning program, in order to reduce the stiffness and soreness that is likely to occur. Particular attention should be given to stretching exercises, which help alleviate the potential joint and muscle problems that seem to be more common in older persons.[15]

A medical examination before starting a conditioning program is essential for the older person. These examinations should continue regularly, probably every year or two, or according to the advice of a physician. This is especially true for any person with a history of illness or cardiac disease.

WRAPPING IT UP

When it comes to exercise, it is important to recognize individual differences. Each individual will have a different degree and kind of physical fitness and will therefore differ in his or her ability to adapt to the demands of a particular strenuous activity. So do not, for example, try to run as fast or as far as your friend until you are ready. Remember, it took you years to get to this stage in life; likewise, it will take you several weeks, or months, or even years to make the changes you want. Don't expect overnight success, and don't expect something for nothing. You are the only one who can do the work required, and you are the one who will get the payoff.

Find a way to enjoy the activities that will improve your physical fitness. Enjoyment is 90 percent psychological. If the activity is really important to you, you will find a way to enjoy it. Make physical fitness and self-improvement a way of life. Become addicted to maintaining your improved self. Try to sell the idea to others, especially those close to you. In this way you will become involved. Don't be discouraged if others let you down, or if you let yourself down now and then. The road to physical fitness and self-improvement may have many stops along the way, and many rough detours. But the pot of gold at the end is worth finding—and you'll know when you've found it.

Notes

1. Laurence Morehouse and Leonard Gross, *Maximum Performance* (New York: Simon and Schuster, 1977), p. 75.
2. Jean Cox Penn, "A Full Gym in Your Home," *Los Angeles Magazine* 24 (January 1979), p. 164.
3. "Health Spas: Svelte For Sale," *Consumer Reports* 43 (August 1978), p. 444.
4. Charles T. Knutzleman and Editors of *Consumer Guide, Rating the Exercises* (New York: William Morrow and Company, Inc., 1978), pp. 264–65.
5. *Ibid.*, pp. 176–78.
6. Herbert A. deVries, *Physiology of Exercise* (Dubuque: Wm. C. Brown Company Publishers, 1974), p. 336.
7. Jack H. Wilmore, *Athletic Training and Physical Fitness* (Boston: Allyn and Bacon, Inc., 1977), p. 193. See also, deVries, *Physiology of Exercise*, p. 365.
8. Wilmore, *Athletic Training and Physical Fitness*, p. 191.
9. *Ibid.*, p. 143.
10. Kenneth C. Lersten, *Physiology and Physical Conditioning* (Palo Alto: Peek Publications, 1974), p. 71.
11. Laurence Morehouse and Leonard Gross, *Total Fitness* (New York: Simon and Schuster, 1975), p. 21.
12. Paul M. Insel and Walton T. Roth, *Health in a Changing Society* (Palo Alto: Mayfield Publishing Company, 1977), p. 108.
13. Lersten, *Physiology and Physical Conditioning*, p. 64.
14. E. Asumssen and P. Mathiasen, "Some Physiologic Functions in Physical Education Students Re-investigated after Twenty-five Years," *Journal of the American Geriatric Society* 10 (1962), pp. 379–87.
15. Wilmore, p. 199.

APPENDIX A

VITAMINS AND MINERALS: FUNCTION, DEFICIENCY CONDITIONS, AND FOOD SOURCES

VITAMINS
(U.S. RDA values are listed in Chapter 4)

	Vitamin	Function	Deficiency condition	Food sources
Fat soluble	Vitamin A (retinal) and provitamin A (α,β,γ-carotene, cryptoxanthin)	1. Adaptation to dim light 2. Promote growth 3. Prevent keratinization of skin and eye 4. Resistance to bacterial infection	1. Night 2. Xerophthalmia 3. Hyperkeratosis 4. Poor growth	Vitamin A Liver Egg yolk Milk, butter Provitamin A ·Sweet potatoes Winter squash Greens Carrots Cantaloupe
	Vitamin D (calciferol)	1. Facilitate absorption of calcium and phosphorus 2. Maintenance of alkaline phosphatase for optimum calcification	1. Rickets 2. Osteomalacia	Vitamin D-fortified milk Eggs Cheese, butter Fish
	Vitamin E (tocopherols)	1. Antioxidant (protects vitamins A and C and unsaturated fatty acids		Vegetable oils Greens
	Vitamin K (phyllo- and farnoquinone)	1. Blood clotting (formation of prothrombin and proconvertin)	1. Hemorrhage	Greens Liver Egg yolks
Water soluble	Thiamin	1. Coenzyme TPP (energy from carbohydrate and fat) 2. Formation of ribose for DNA and RNA (transketolase) 3. Conversion of tryptophan to niacin	1. Beriberi	Meat Whole grain and enriched cereals Milk Legumes
	Riboflavin	1. FMN and FAD for releasing energy 2. Conversion of tryptophan to niacin	1. Ariboflavinosis	Milk Green vegetables Fish, meat, eggs
	Niacin	1. NAD and NADP to release energy 2. Glycolysis 3. Fatty acid synthesis	1. Pellagra	Meat, poultry, fish Peanut butter Whole grain and enriched cereals Greens

SOURCE: Fredrick J. Stare and Margaret McWilliams, *Living Nutrition.* Copyright © 1973 by John Wiley & Sons, Inc. Reprinted by permission of John Wiley & Sons, Inc.

VITAMINS

Vitamin	Function	Deficiency condition	Food sources
Vitamin B$_6$ (pyridoxine)	1. Transamination and deamination of amino acids 2. Porphyrin synthesis (for hemoglobin) 3. Conversion of tryptophan to niacin 4. Energy from glycogen 5. Formation of histamine, serotonin, norepinephrine		Meats Bananas Whole grain cereals Lima beans Cabbage Potatoes Spinach
Pantothenic acid	1. CoA component (transfer 2 carbon fragments to release energy) 2. Porphyrin synthesis (hemoglobin formation) 3. Cholesterol and steroid formation		Organ meats Whole grain cereal
Biotin	1. Release energy from carbohydrate 2. Fatty acid metabolism 3. Deamination of protein		Egg yolks Milk Organ meats Cereals Legumes Nuts
Folacin (folic acid, pteroylglutamic acid)	1. Transfer of single carbon units 2. Coenzyme in synthesis of: guanine and adenine; thymine; choline; amino acids; porphyrin	1. Macrocytic anemia	Greens Mushrooms Liver Kidney
Vitamin B$_{12}$ (cobalamin)	1. Maturation of red blood cells 2. Carbohydrate metabolism for energy for central nervous system 3. Formation of single carbon radicals 4. Conversion of folinic acid to folacin	1. Pernicious anemia	Animal foods
Ascorbic acid (vitamin C)	Formation of collagen 2. Utilization of calcium in bones and teeth 3. Elasticity and strength of capillaries 4. Conversion of folinic acid to folacin	1. Scurvy	Citrus fruits Strawberries Papayas Broccoli Cabbage Tomatoes Potatoes

MINERALS
(U.S. RDA values are listed in Chapter 4)

Mineral	Functions	Food sources
Calcium	1. Bone formation, maintenance, and growth 2. Tooth formation 3. Blood clot formation 4. Activation of pancreatic lipase 5. Absorption of vitamin B_{12} 6. Contraction of muscle	Milk, cheese, puddings, custards, chocolate beverages Fish with bones, including salmon Greens Broccoli
Chloride	1. Component of hydrochloric acid 2. Maintenance of proper osmotic pressure 3. Acid-base balance	Table salt Meats Milk Eggs
Cobalt	1. Part of vitamin B_{12} molecule	Organ meats Meats
Copper	1. Catalyst for hemoglobin formation 2. Formation of elastin (connective tissue) 3. Release of energy (in cytochrome oxidase and catalase) 4. Formation of melanin (pigment) 5. Formation of phospholipids for myelin sheath of nerves	Cereals Nuts Legumes Liver Shellfish Grapes Meats
Fluoride	1. Strengthen bones and teeth	Fluoridated water
Iodine	1. Component of thyroxine and tri-iodo-thyronine	Iodized salt Fish (salt water and anadromous)
Iron	1. Component of hemoglobin 2. Component of myoglobin 3. Component of cytochromes, cytochrome oxidase, catalase, peroxidase 4. Component of myeloperoxidase	Meats Heart, liver Clams Oysters Lima beans Spinach Dates, dried fruits Nuts Enriched and whole grain cereals

MINERALS

Mineral	Functions	Food sources
Magnesium	1. Catalyze ATP ↔ ADP 2. Conduct nerve impulses 3. Retention of calcium in teeth 4. Adjust to cold environment	Milk Green vegetables Nuts Breads and cereals
Manganese	1. Bone development 2. Component of arginase 3. Promotes thiamin storage	Cereals Legumes
Molybdenum	1. Component of xanthine oxidase 2. Component of aldehyde oxidase	

Phosphorus	1. Bone formation, maintenance, and growth
	2. Tooth formation
	3. Component of DNA and RNA
	4. Component of ADP and ATP
	5. Fatty acid transport
	6. Acid-base balance
	7. Component of TPP
		Organic
		  Meats, poultry, and fish
		Inorganic
		  Milk, fruits and
		    vegetables

Potassium	1. Maintenance of osmotic pressure 2. Acid-base balance 3. Transmission of nerve impulses 4. Catalyst in energy metabolism 5. Formation of proteins 6. Formation of glycogen	Orange juice Dried fruits Bananas Potatoes Coffee
Selenium	1. Antioxidant	
Sodium	1. Maintenance of osmotic pressure 2. Acid-base balance 3. Relaxation of muscles 4. Absorption of glucose 5. Transmission of nerve impulses	Table salt Salted meats Milk
Sulfur	1. Component of thiamin 2. Component of some proteins (hair, nails, skin)	Meats Milk and cheese Eggs Legumes Nuts
Zinc	1. Component of carboxypeptidase 2. Component of carbonic anhydrase	Whole-grain cereals Meats Legumes

APPENDIX B

Heart Rate Count Chart

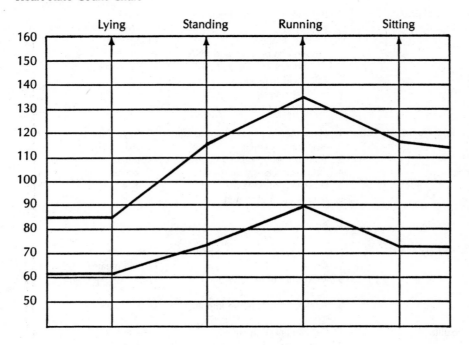

This chart illustrates the average number of heart beats per minute required by the human body for different routine activities. The upper line shows a typical example of the extra work that the heart has to do when a person is not physically fit. The lower line shows the results of an average person who engages in a regular, vigorous exercise program. Following the directions below, fill in a line showing how your heart beat reacts to each activity. Indicate the number of beats for each activity to the left of the numbered statement.

_____ 1. Rest in a lying position for 5 minutes, take your pulse for 60 seconds and record.

_____ 2. Stand up, take pulse immediately for 10 seconds and multiply by 6 (to get 60 seconds). A physically fit person will have no more than a 10-second difference from the resting rate.*

_____ 3. Run in place briskly for 1 minute, sit down and immediately take your pulse for 10 seconds and multiply by 6. See rating:

Rating of pulse rate after running in place.†

84–96 beats . . . Very good	138–149 beats . . . Below average
102–114 beats . . . Above average	150–161 beats . . . Poor
120–132 beats . . . Average	162+ beats . . . Very poor

_____ 4. Sit down for a minute, count pulse for 10 seconds. (Pulse should not exceed 110.)

_____ 5. After running in place 1 minute, a physically fit person should be able to recover to standing pulse rate in 5 minutes or less. Count your pulse during the first 10 seconds of each minute until it is equal to or lower than your standing pulse (2). In totaling the recovery time, be sure to add the "sitting minute" in 4.

*Herbert A. deVries, *Physiology of Exercise* (Dubuque: Wm. C. Brown Company, 1976), p. 104.
†Curtis Mitchess, *The Perfect Exercise* (New York: Simon and Schuster, 1976), p. 57.

APPENDIX C

PULSE RATE TRAINING ZONES
(Ten-second counts in parentheses)

Age	Maximum pulse rate attainable (220 − age)	Training limits	
		Upper 85% of maximum	Lower 70% of maximum
14	206	175 (29)	144 (24)
16	204	173 (29)	143 (24)
18	202	171 (29)	141 (24)
20	200	170 (28)	140 (23)
22	198	168 (28)	139 (23)
24	196	167 (28)	137 (23)
26	194	165 (27)	136 (23)
28	192	163 (27)	134 (22)
30	190	162 (27)	133 (22)
32	188	160 (27)	132 (22)
34	186	158 (26)	130 (22)
36	184	156 (26)	129 (21)
38	182	155 (26)	127 (21)
40	180	153 (26)	126 (21)

SOURCE: Lenore R. Zohman, *Beyond Diet . . . Exercise your Way to Fitness and Heart Health* (CPC International, Inc., 1974), p. 15.

APPENDIX D

Weight-Training Record Sheet

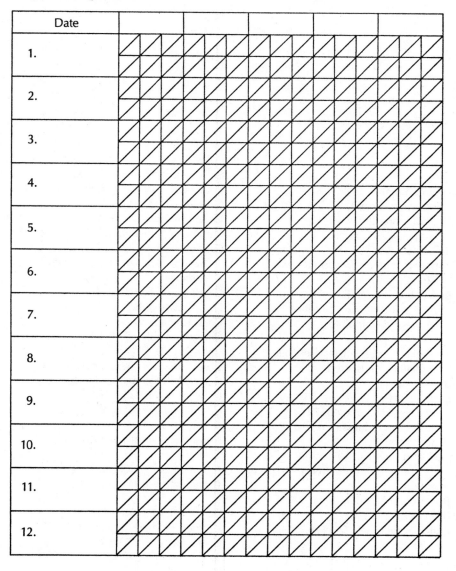

Date					
1.					
2.					
3.					
4.					
5.					
6.					
7.					
8.					
9.					
10.					
11.					
12.					

INDEX